Cognitive Behaviour Therapy

An Introduction to Theory and Practice

Cognitive Behaviour Therapy

An Introduction to Theory and Practice

Edited by

Sue Marshall

Clinical Psychologist
The Black Country Mental Health Trust

and

John Turnbull

Nursing Officer
(Learning Disabilities)
Department of Health

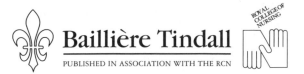

Baillière Tindall

PUBLISHED IN ASSOCIATION WITH THE RCN

London   Philadelphia   Toronto   Sydney   Tokyo

Baillière Tindall 24–28 Oval Road
London NW1 7DX

The Curtis Center
Independence Square West
Philadelphia, PA 19106-3399, USA

Harcourt Brace & Company
55 Horner Avenue
Toronto, Ontario, M8Z 4X6, Canada

Harcourt Brace & Company, Australia
30–52 Smidmore Street
Marrickville
NSW 2204, Australia

Harcourt Brace & Company, Japan
Ichibancho Central Building
Chiyoda-ku, Tokyo 102, Japan

A catalogue record for this book is available from the British Library

ISBN 0-7020-1967-4

Typeset by Paston Press Ltd, Loddon, Norfolk
Printed and bound in Great Britain by WBC, Bridgend, Mid Glamorgan

Contents

Contributors

Althea Allison, MA Health Care Ethics, BSc Hons Nursing Studies, RMN, CPN, RCNT/FETC, RNT/Cert Ed, is Lecturer in Community Studies and Course Leader for Community Mental Health Nursing, Department of Community Studies, University of Reading (UK).

Andy Farrington, MA, BA(Hons), Hon PGDip (Prague), RMN, Cert BPsychotherapy, Teaching Cert, is Senior Research Fellow in Nursing, Department of Nursing and Midwifery, De Montfort University, Leicester (UK).

Sue Marshall, MPhil, BA(Hons) RGN is a Clinical Psychologist with The Black Country Mental Health Trust and Honorary Lecturer at The University of Birmingham (UK).

Andrew Stevens, MSc Clinical Psychology, BSc, is Clinical Psychologist with Northampton Healthcare Community NHS Trust.

Anni Telford, MA, Hon PGDip (Prague), RMN, Cert Cog Psych, Cert BPsychotherapy, Cert Ed, Cert R.E.T, is Head of Counselling and Psychotherapy, Unit for Counselling Practice and Research, School of Education and Social Science, University of Derby (UK).

John Turnbull, MSc, BA, RNMH, is a Nursing Officer (Learning Disabilities) at the Department of Health and Honorary Lecturer at the University of Reading (UK).

SECTION 1

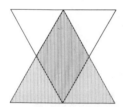

The Principles of Cognitive Behaviour Therapy

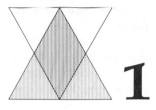 **1**

Introduction
The aims of this book and how to use it

John Turnbull and Sue Marshall

Aims

Cognitive behaviour therapy is a well-researched and proven approach to psychological problems that has contributed immensely to the improvement of people's lifestyles. It has rapidly become the treatment of choice for more common mental health problems such as depression and is achieving growing success in contributing to people's recovery from physical health problems as well as helping to improve their close relationships. At the same time, a growing number of professionals from different backgrounds are encountering these benefits. Many of these professionals will already have acquired skills in applying cognitive behaviour therapy with their own clients, whilst others will have recognised similarities between this approach and their own methods of helping people.

Although the value of cognitive behaviour therapy is implied throughout this book, our central aim is to clarify the principal elements of its approach and to encourage improvements in practice. Therefore, the chapters that follow will avoid the usual approach of describing the disorders to which cognitive behaviour therapy is applied. Instead, the contributors will present their chapters in a way that enables you to establish the key elements of practice, to recognise the limits of your current competence and to identify ways in which your practice could be improved. Each chapter will set out its own objectives, but a standard format has been used to provide both continuity and to reflect the importance we attach to four principal themes. Firstly, each chapter will clearly establish the strategies that need to be employed at a particular stage in the therapeutic process. Secondly, contributors will consider the development of the relationship between the therapist and the client. Thirdly, they will demonstrate what can be done when things fail to go according to plan. Finally, each of the contributors has been asked to address the issue of supervision of practice as being an important means of demonstrating accountability.

Ultimately, the success of this approach will rest with you and we do not claim that this book alone will enable you to become totally proficient in the practice of cognitive behaviour therapy. However, we hope that the style and structure of the book will provide an important platform for your development.

With this is mind, we would now ask you to complete an exercise which will be repeated at the end of the book. The purpose is to help you clarify your current thoughts about your role as a helper.

Self-assessment exercise

This exercise has been prepared to give you an opportunity to reflect on your skills as a cognitive behaviour therapist. In completing the exercise you need to be honest about your current level of competence. It is probably a good idea to discuss your response to the various questions with someone you know well and who is familiar with your clinical work.

This assessment is not a standardised tool – it is simply a guideline to help you be reflective in your practice.

1. Think about someone you know who is an example of a competent cognitive behaviour therapist. Describe the skills and knowledge they have. If you cannot summarize these, then ask the person to do it with you. Try to identify which characteristics are 'skills' and which are 'knowledge'.
2. Using the list as a guide, consider which of these characteristics you currently have. On a scale of 1–10 think what you would score for each of them (1 = do not have, 10 = feel fully competent).
3. Ask for a client's permission to tape a session of therapy and use the tape to assess yourself on the characteristics you have identified as features of a skilled therapist. It is a good idea to use tapes as part of your supervision to help you to identify areas of strength and need in your practice.

Structure

The aim of the cognitive behaviour therapist is to apply the underlying principles of the approach through a range of strategies, which are carefully selected to meet the individual needs of the client. The specific strategies that are employed can be found in Section 2, which forms the most substantial part of this book. The chapters within that section take you through the initial stage of assessment to the final stage of discharging the client. However, we should remember that the therapeutic process includes two people: the client and the therapist. Section 2 can deal only with the part of therapy that the client experiences. In reality the therapeutic process begins before the client comes through your door. Prior to this, the process will be influenced by your expectations, the preparation you have had for your role and the culture within which you practise. It will also be affected by the client's expectations and needs. Therefore, Section 1 will set out the main issues that affect your practice, including a description of the principles that underpin the cognitive behavioural approach. Similarly, when the client has been discharged and disappears through your office door, the therapeutic process continues by means of your own reflection on this experience and, hopefully, an improvement in practice. Therefore, Section 3 will focus on ways in which personal and professional growth can be encouraged.

First principles

In the next chapter, we will discuss in more detail some of the issues that go to the heart of current professional practice. Many of these issues are concerned with the need for professionals to be both fit for purpose and fit for practice. In practical terms, this means having a clear idea of the needs of people and being able to meet these needs by consistently applying the appropriate level of skill.

Therefore, we shall begin chapter two by looking at the types of need which can be met by the cognitive behavioural approach. In an era in which medicine has dominated professional practice and the expectations of the general public, we will set cognitive behaviour therapy along a continuum of help which will demonstrate its relevance to a range of human problems. Within a context of increasing pressure on budgets, managers are posing many questions that will ultimately result in the need to target scarce expertise. An important question, therefore, is whether it is possible to identify the point at which professional practice should take over from either self-help or the help that is offered by non-professionals, either paid or unpaid. Questions such as these have led to the development of evidence-based training in which the demonstration of competence appears to be valued more than the title or qualification possessed by an individual worker. Whereas this has raised anxieties in the minds of many professionals, others have seen this move as a way of strengthening their practice: after all, competence is a threat to incompetent practice, not professional preparation.

Moving on from the factors that influence the thinking of professionals, the client will also come to therapy with their own expectations. It is firstly important to recognise that cognitive behaviour therapy is being practised against a background in which people have generally been encouraged to take increasing responsibility for their actions. On a positive note, this emphasis on individuality can lead to increasing wealth and feelings of personal freedom. The negative side of the situation can be an emphasis on independence rather than individuality. In turn, this can lead to a severance of important relationships. Secondly, anyone who cannot achieve the dream of personal expression could be left with feelings of inadequacy, believing that they only have themselves to blame for their distress. In many instances, nothing could be further from the truth.

If we transfer the emphasis on self-management to the arena of health care, a similar pattern emerges. The public now has access to considerable amounts of literature and advice on improving their health. Furthermore, the involvement of the person in their own health services has been encouraged by initiatives such as the Patients' Charter (Department of Health 1991). The inclusion of people in their own care and the formation of partnerships with health professionals is an idea that seems to make so much sense that it is difficult to envisage a time when professionals resisted it. Despite this belief, it is not always easy to implement it. As far as cognitive behaviour therapy is concerned, its principles demand the level of partnership that other aspects of health care would envy. This partnership approach is reflected in both the relationships that therapists form with their clients as well as the specific strategies employed and is a feature upon which the following chapter as well as the rest of the book will place great emphasis.

The inclusion of people in their own therapy is not simply carried out because it is fashionable. It is derived from the view of people and the origins of their problems, which the cognitive behaviour therapist holds. In Chapter 3, Sue Marshall elaborates on this by tracing the development of the cognitive behavioural approach. Although cognitive behaviour therapy is an approach drawn from a range of psychological theories and techniques, its distinctive feature is the view of people as being active seekers, selectors and interpreters of experiences. This leads to the goal of therapy as being one which encourages people to become their own therapist. Reviewing the research literature, Sue Marshall shows how people develop their own unique ways of thinking about the world. This enables people to anticipate events by constructing hypotheses about how people might behave as well as the reasons for this. This creativity is central to the survival of the human race but, on an individual level, it can create difficulties for some. People will sometimes develop irrational beliefs about the behaviour of others or themselves, which can interfere with normal functioning and result in distress. Cognitive behaviour therapists therefore seek to enable individuals to modify their thoughts and beliefs, which in turn will improve performance and alleviate distress.

Applying first principles

The application of the principles discussed in the first three chapters is the subject of Section 2. The three chapters presented here will deal with the time that the client spends in therapy. In Chapter 4, Andy Farrington and Anni Telford present assessment as the essential first step in therapy, during which a therapeutic relationship is established. Many people will come into this first stage of therapy after trying and probably failing to help themselves. Therefore, confidence will be low. Andy Farrington and Anni Telford cover in detail the specific actions that need to be taken by the therapist to develop trust and confidence in the therapist and the therapy itself. The important point is made that, in order to encourage a trusting relationship, the skilled therapist will not substitute the interview for checklists. This relationship can be helped by establishing solid ground rules for sessions at an early stage, and clarifying expectations about the responsibilities of both therapist and client.

Although assessment is not a 'one-off' procedure, and constant evaluation and clarification of information is required, Andy Farrington and Anni Telford provide a sound framework for obtaining the necessary information. The first thing to establish is precisely what problems are being caused by the behaviour of the client. What are the consequences of this behaviour continuing or discontinuing? Behaviour can be seen in terms of excesses, deficits or assets. It is also important to gauge the frequency, intensity and duration of the behaviour that is responsible for feelings of distress. It is also important to assess the client's own motivation to change. This can be a crucial factor: as Andy Farrington and Anni Telford point out, it is always possible to change things, but will it be worth the effort as far as the client is concerned?

Since cognitive behaviour therapy centres its approach on the thoughts and beliefs of the client, this chapter will describe a range of strategies to help the client and therapist to access them. Imaginal techniques, setting behavioural tasks to help generate and capture thoughts, video tests and essay writing are amongst some of the methods that help to formulate a hypothesis about the origins of the client's problem.

In anticipation of the following chapter, Andy Farrington and Anni Telford conclude by stressing the importance of setting goals for the problems that have been identified. Decisions will need to be made with the client about targets for their performance, remembering that, in these early stages, confidence may not be high. Decisions will also need to be taken concerning the appropriateness of other approaches, for example, relaxation or the use of co-therapists. If things go well, the client and therapist should be well prepared for the subsequent sessions in which strategies to change the client's cognitions and behaviour will be employed.

A framework for intervention

In Chapter 5, Andrew Stevens begins by reiterating the importance of giving the client clear explanations in order to maintain their commitment and clarify expectations. This paves the way for the client's increasing participation in their own therapy. Andrew Stevens also suggests additional ways in which the therapist can 'sell the rationale' of cognitive behaviour therapy through the use of written information.

The bulk of this chapter, however, is concerned with employing the more active components of therapy. This is the stage at which the client is taught to recognise and modify the thoughts and beliefs that form the basis for the problem. Using real-life examples, Andrew Stevens shows how the use of Socratic questioning can encourage the client to reflect upon the impact of their cognitions. This technique is particularly important as it challenges the client without threatening their growing, but fragile, confidence.

Learning to replace unhelpful cognitions within the therapist's office will not, of course, be sufficient to bring about improvements. Cognitive behavioural therapy depends for its success on employing **behavioural** as well as **cognitive** strategies. Building upon the strategies already introduced in Chapter 4, Andrew Stevens continues to recommend the setting of achievable tasks that the client can practice. Depending upon the problem, he also describes specific measures that can be employed to reinforce learning. Phobic clients, for example, will benefit from gradual exposure to the object of their problem. Clients who may believe certain experiences will be too distressing for them, such as job interviews, can be taught to construct hierarchies of tasks through which practice can lead to increased confidence. Some clients may need to learn specific interpersonal or communication skills to help develop their relationships with their partner or family. Acquiring time management or organisational skills can also contribute to alleviating feelings of stress at work.

Things will go wrong at every stage of the process of therapy. Difficulties at this stage are likely to be put right by clarifying the client's understanding and challenging cognitions the client may have about the therapy itself. Opportunities still exist to go back one stage and reformulate the problem.

Handing over

In the final chapter of this section, Anni Telford and Andy Farrington return to consider the issue of handing over the therapy to the client. Although each stage of the process of therapy is important, this is the stage by which the client will have fully developed the insight into the nature of their difficulties and possesses the skills to deal with them. The outcome will be a client who has taken on the skills of the therapist and can apply them to a range of settings.

The specific strategies described in this chapter are those that ensure that the client will be able to apply their learning. Whilst the client is still in a relatively safe environment, the therapist will need to help the client anticipate failure. By using self-instruction and the framework of enquiry introduced to them in previous stages, the client can rehearse their response.

As the client develops these skills and begins to use them, there will be important implications for people such as family and friends. Anni Telford and Andy Farrington discuss the possibility of enlisting the help of these people as 'co-therapists'. It will also be important to consider the impact of the changes in the client upon those who are close to them. Any misunderstanding may jeopardise the gains the client has made. The therapist will need to discuss these changes with them.

Eventually the decision must be taken to discharge the client. It is important that this decision is seen as one which ends a **stage** in the process of therapy. Cognitive behaviour therapy is a self-management approach in which the client is empowered through the learning of techniques to become their own therapist. Discharge is therefore the beginning of real growth for the person.

An ethical framework

Ethical issues are central to the practice of every professional, no matter what their practice or choice of therapeutic approach. Such is the importance that we attach to these issues, that we have included a separate chapter to help you understand the principles underlying sound ethical practice and to help you overcome the dilemmas you will encounter. Far from providing a strait-jacket to confine the limits to our practice, Chapter 7 will show how ethical principles exist to help us improve our it.

In Chapter 7, Althea Allison firstly points out that cognitive behaviour therapy is a powerful process that seeks to change thoughts and behaviour. This places responsibilities upon the therapist, which can be exercised through the use of sound reasoning and respect for the individual client. As the chapters on practice issues will point out, some of the tasks which clients will be asked to carry out will be uncomfortable. The distress that this may cause might appear to conflict with the therapist's overall commitment to avoid harm to the individual. Therefore, it is crucial that the therapist is able to plan and implement the specific techniques of therapy in a deliberate manner in order ultimately to bring about positive and long-lasting change in the individual. It is also crucial that the relationship between the therapist and the client is one that instils trust and reassurance. Whereas these are characteristics that might be the outcome of many types of social relationships, Althea Allison stresses, the therapist does not have the luxury of time nor the obligation to develop this type of closeness with the client. The trust that arises from the client–therapist relationship is based upon the ethical principles of accepting each person unconditionally. This can be difficult in cases in which the client has acted in ways which we would normally disapprove of, such as wife beating.

The chapter concludes by encouraging us to recognise the limits of our knowledge. This places obligations on us to take responsibilities for our own personal and professional development which is the subject of the final section.

Practice-based development

Since this book uses the generic term 'therapist' to describe the person using cognitive behaviour therapy, it cannot be assumed that all practitioners will come from the same background and with the same knowledge. Section 3 stresses the need for any therapist, whatever his or her background, to continue to develop their skills. It will differ from the rest of the book by setting out a series of exercises which will provide a framework to help you fulfil this obligation.

In the same way that we would expect our clients to take forward the skills they have learnt, it should also represent the beginning of another stage for the therapist. We would therefore hope that the framework provided in the final chapter is one to which you will return each time one of your clients is discharged.

Good luck.

Reference

Department of Health. **The Patient's Charter**. London: Department of Health.

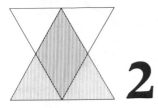

2

The Context of Therapy

John Turnbull

Key issues

- Uniqueness of individual experience
- Key factors influencing therapeutic practice
- Understanding the nature of needs
- Needs of the therapist

Quote – John Turnbull

Overview

Cognitive behaviour therapy is an approach to helping people cope more effectively with problems by equipping them with a framework of thinking and behaving, which enables them to lead more fulfilling lives. The essential components of this approach are based on a belief that the world is experienced differently by each person. Therefore, the individual will develop his or her own unique sets of beliefs, which, in turn, will influence how events are interpreted and, ultimately, how the person will act. This is a process that applies equally to the therapist as it does to the client seeking help.

11

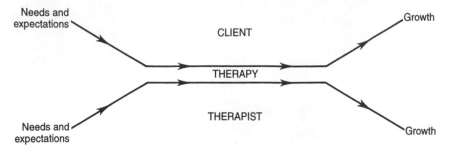

Figure 2.1   Model of the therapeutic process.

The uniqueness of this experience forms a central theme within this book and is the focus of this chapter. From your own point of view, this chapter will set out the key factors that are currently influencing therapeutic practice. It will also show how these experiences should be understood within the context of the therapeutic process. As Figure 2.1 illustrates, this process can be seen as being influenced by distinctive but parallel types of events that take place both before and after the actual encounter between the client and therapist. Using this as a model, the aim of this chapter is to improve your practice by discussing the issues relating specifically to the early stage of the therapeutic process. The needs and expectations of both the client and therapist will be discussed. For example, it will address the question of how we should understand the nature of the needs of people. In turn, this will influence how assessment of these needs should be undertaken. Finally, the chapter will discuss the needs of the therapist in the organisational context in which he or she works.

First principles

To begin with, let us examine the factors that give rise to the need for help. Imagine the situation of a man in his early thirties coming to you for help. He has recently moved into the area from a town 50 miles away with his family following a job promotion. He tells you that he is having difficulty sleeping, he experiences panic attacks, he has lost confidence and finds it difficult to concentrate. He also feels depressed: he has moved home before as a result of a change in job and has always managed to settle in well and make friends. He has been feeling this way despite the efforts of his wife, and talking to some of his friends and colleagues he has left behind.

During the interview with him, you ask him if he has any idea why he is experiencing his symptoms. 'I don't really know', he says. 'I must be going mad. I went to the doctor because I thought it might be a brain tumour or something like that. He said I should come and see you ... I must really be in trouble if I have to see you ... I can't understand it ... I've got the chance of a lifetime and I'm blowing it. I've moved before and thing's went okay ... it should be the same this time ... what am I doing wrong?'

This brief example introduces us to many of the ideas to be discussed in this chapter. These might be summarised as follows:

- Need arises out of the discrepancy between the person's external and internal environment.
- The external environment can influence the person's expectations of the therapeutic process.
- The goal of cognitive behaviour therapy is to bring about self-directed change through the medium of the partnership between the person and therapist.

Using the example given above, let us examine these issues in more detail.

Understanding human needs

First of all, let us consider the example in terms of the needs of people. People generally seek to achieve the right 'fit' between themselves and their environment. By environment, we should think of anything other than the individual, such as his or her family, friends, job and surroundings. This 'person-context fit' is achieved when the person minimises the effects of the demands made by the environment as well as strengthens his or her skills and abilities. This is shown in a diagramatic format in Figure 2.2. Here, the inner circle represents the individual and his or her skills, beliefs and personal characteristics. The outer circle represents the environment and the people in it. Any progress towards achieving the right fit is felt when the inner circle moves to fill up more of the space between itself and the outer circle.

Many things in life rarely remain the same. Therefore, in terms of the diagram, we cannot expect the environment to stay where it is. Consider the example of a man who loses his job. Figure 2.3 shows the result. The environment has moved to create a gap, or an area of need. The man feels intensely angry and needs help from you to get him back on his feet and fill the gap by getting another job.

Imagine, however, that instead of becoming angry because he lost his job, the man had lost his job because he became angry. In terms of the diagram, the effect would be the same in that a gap would appear. However, your approach to helping him fill this gap would change.

Let us return to the example given earlier in the chapter and consider it in the light of the diagrams you have just seen. What do you consider to be

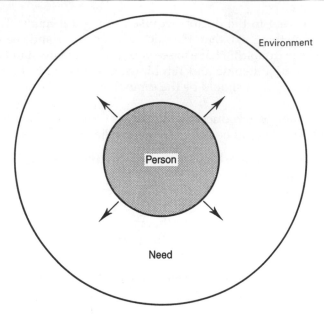

Figure 2.2   The person-context 'fit'.

the causes of the person's feelings? Looking at the environment, this has clearly changed. Not only have the physical surroundings changed, but the man's job is different and he has new colleagues. However, as he has said himself, he has coped with this before and any assessment should investigate precisely what steps he took before. One reason for his current distress could simply be that he lacks practice. Further therapy sessions might include thinking more deliberately about creating opportunities to become integrated into his new community. Another reason might be to examine in more detail the expectations of the man prior to moving. From some of his statements we can already see that he has some fixed ideas about how the world should be. It is possible that his expectations that things would be the same were unrealistic? In one way, his success in the past has created the conditions for future disappointments. Perhaps the way forward in therapy should be to focus on encouraging a more flexible thinking style.

Whereas this model of human need will help the therapist understand the nature of his or her practice, it will also help us to begin to clarify the expectations of the client. Looking back at some of the statements made by the man, we notice that he imagined his symptoms to be the result of a physical cause, namely a brain tumour. It is not unusual for many people to think of their problems in terms of an illness. Some of this is the result of the physical symptoms that people experience, even in

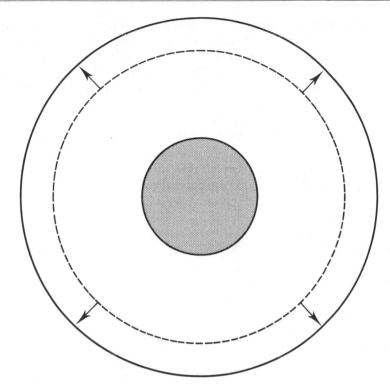

Figure 2.3   The creation of need.

situations in which the cause is psychological, such as increased heart rate or headaches. However, this is also the result of the dominance of a medical style of thinking. This thinking leads people to look for a name or a diagnosis of the problem. Kahn and Earle (1982) have described this as a belief in 'the magic of naming' (p. 49), as if giving a problem a name can, somehow, bring it under control. A diagnosis also implies a cure and people may arrive in the therapist's office with the expectation that they will receive something that will enable them to become the same as they were before the problem began. How should we respond if the man in the earlier example had such beliefs? He may expect his lifestyle prior to moving home to suddenly return as a result of therapy. The job of the therapist is to persuade him that therapy will help him to respond more flexibly rather than restore what existed beforehand.

This may help to give the client a clearer view of what might happen at the end of therapy. However, the expectations raised by a medically dominated thinking style are worth considering for a little longer to help us appreciate the breadth of problems amenable to the cognitive behavioural approach.

The expectation of a return to normal functioning is accurate in cases which genuinely require a medical approach. The entry of bacteria into the body will result in an infection. Applying antibiotics to remove the cause of the problem will result in the absence of infection and the body will return to its normal state. Other cases may require a medical contribution but cannot be seen in precisely the same way. For example, someone who experiences a stroke will show physical symptoms such as a loss of speech or mobility. Perfect health cannot, however, be restored even though physiotherapy may alleviate some of the physical symptoms. Adaptations to the person's home will also help to eliminate areas of need. Cognitive behaviour therapy can be particularly useful here in helping the person to adjust their own expectations, especially to accept that things cannot be how they were prior to the stroke.

The example of a stroke is one in which the person is in a state of deprivation. This means that they have suffered a loss of skills. Cognitive behaviour therapy helps them adjust to this loss. Other types of problems amenable to cognitive behaviour therapy include those in which the person is said to be in a state of 'privation'. In other words, problems are caused because the person lacks skills. Consider problems that arise within family relationships. These problems can often be attributed to a lack of skills in communication and negotiation. Similarly, people experiencing problems of self-control may never have learned problem-solving or relaxation techniques. The goal of cognitive behaviour therapy in these cases would be to help people acquire these skills and to modify their interpretation of situations.

To summarise, people's problems arise when needs cannot be met. Need can be seen as a discrepancy between a person's internal and external environment. This balance can be upset by the impact of a loss or by a lack of adjustment on the part of the individual. In order for cognitive behaviour therapy to be successful, this must be clearly understood by the client. The therapist also benefits from this model of need as it helps him or her appreciate the types of problems to which cognitive behaviour therapy is amenable.

Role expectations

Not only will expectations be affected by the way the client and the therapist view the therapy itself, they will also be affected by their view of their respective roles. What are the influences that are at work here? Returning to the example of the man who has moved home, we can pick up some useful clues. Once he began to experience problems, we know that he looked to his wife and former colleagues for help. Like many other people, he may also have tried to cope with the problem himself. Clearly recognising no improvement, he consulted his doctor who then referred him on to the therapist. What should we make of his reaction to this? If you remember, he stated that 'I really must be in trouble if I have to see you'.

The man's reaction probably typifies the general view that there exists a hierarchy of expertise, beginning with oneself and ending with an expert. This traditional view is represented by the direction of the arrow shown in the diagram in Figure 2.4 (p. 23). This presents several difficulties for the cognitive behaviour therapist. Firstly, it can compromise the partnership that needs to exist between him or herself and the client. Even though the client may recognise the need to play a role in their own therapy, it may diminish the value they attach to their contribution. It also has an impact upon the therapist by influencing the way they think about the contribution of the professional and the way their skills are deployed within services. This will be discussed later. From the client's point of view, are there any forces working towards changing this view?

The context in which therapy is sought out and provided is changing. To a great extent this is being influenced by the way individuals are being encouraged to see their role. This has been reinforced by key policy documents such as The Patients' Charter (Department of Health 1991), which, for the first time, has given the public a role in respect of the health and social services they receive. This role includes the following elements:

- To take part in the assessment of their needs.
- To raise their expectations of what services could offer and how they could be delivered in order to influence service quality.
- To participate in the evaluation of service quality.
- To use information given on health and social care services in order to make informed choices.

Although the extent to which the public have been proactive in exercising their role might be argued about, their influence has been felt. Making complaints, for example, is seen as a way in which feedback can help services become more user centred. The inclusion of service users and their carers is becoming more commonplace in the strategic planning of services, and in the training and education of professional staff. Surveys of user satisfaction is also a valuable means of evaluating aspects of service provision. On an individual level, this change would include expectations of the person being fully involved as an equal partner in their treatment and care.

In addition to the roles listed earlier, there is another role that is more implicit in the health service reforms. This is an expectation that people should become more self-reliant and will take steps to promote their own well-being. One of the ways that this expectation is communicated is through the financial assessments undertaken when applications for residential or nursing home placements are made. People are now expected to make a contribution to their own care if they have the resources. The implication is that people should act responsibly during their working life in order to make provision for their care later in life.

Another major initiative that has encouraged people to take steps to improve their quality of life came through the launching of the Government's 'Health of the Nation' white paper in 1992 (Department of Health 1992). Like the Patient's Charter, the Health of the Nation has become a major plank of current policy. Unlike other health strategies, the Health of the Nation sets out specific targets for achievement for the whole nation in five key areas. Significantly, as far as this book is concerned, one of the key areas is mental health. The Health of the Nation strategy and subsequent initiatives in the area makes it clear that health is everyone's responsibility.

In view of this discussion, has the required change been achieved? Are people more prepared to look for alternatives to professional help? Has it resulted in greater partnership with professional staff? There is no doubt that people now have greater access to information concerning their own health. The same is also true concerning personal relationships and aspects of psychological well-being. Evidence for improvement is more difficult to find. Many people appear to have heeded the advice on fitness. Evidence for improved mental health and relationships are more difficult to establish.

As far as improved partnership between professionals and the public is concerned, expectations of professional performance appear to have increased. For example, general practitioners report increasing demands upon their services out of surgery hours. In the light of this, any change in the expectations and actions of clients at an individual level appears to rely upon the relationship that is established between the client and the therapist during the process of therapy. Although this is an aspect of the therapeutic process that will be discussed by each contributor in subsequent chapters, some general points will be made now.

The therapeutic relationship

A great deal of attention in the academic literature has focused on the nature of the relationship between the client and therapist. This is often described as a partnership or even an alliance (Horvath and Greenberg 1993). Many of the answers to the questions raised about the significance of this relationship can be found first of all by looking at the goals of therapy itself. Barker (1989) points out that the word therapy is derived from the Greek word *therapeutike*, meaning the art of healing. Given our previous discussion about the needs of people, we can see how the goals of cognitive behaviour therapy can be likened to this healing process. The focus on helping people to adjust implies that therapy is concerned with both aims and outcomes. In other words, there must be a deliberate effort made by a person to bring about learning and adjustment to the demands of the environment. This deliberate action is composed of specific techniques which are the subject of the chapters in Section 2.

However, the success of these techniques has been found to depend upon other aspects of the process, such as the nature of the relationship between the client and therapist. In discussing the nature of this relationship, Cain (1995) firstly distinguishes all professional relationships from social relationships. Any relationship between a professional and his or her client is essentially a contractual one in which the professional owes the client a duty of care. In addition to these legal constraints, professional codes of conduct will also prohibit certain types of behaviour, such as sexual intimacy, even though the client may consent. This type of relationship is quite different from social relationships, such as friendship. As Cain points out, social relationships are formed on the basis of two people liking each other and finding their friendship mutually beneficial. Whereas the client and therapist may come to like each other, this is a by-product of the relationship and not a necessary condition for therapy to succeed. Furthermore, even though the therapist might be expected to learn from the therapeutic encounter, the focus is on benefiting the client. In other words, the therapist might gain from the relationship but should never give their services in the expectation of gaining.

The contributors to Section 2 point out that the relationship between client and therapist will change as they progress through the stages of therapy. In his discussion of relationships, Cain also sees it as a dynamic process. Perhaps unexpectedly, Cain firstly proposes that relationships can display aspects of paternalism. Paternalism is usually associated with outmoded forms of care in which information is withheld from the client, thus limiting the exercise of choice. However, Cain points out that the therapist may sometimes need to coerce the client into carrying out actions which he or she will find unpleasant in order that progress can ultimately be made. This is something that may often be required early in therapy when the client may not be in a position to make choices. Although this action will be based upon the ethical principles of beneficence (see Chapter 7), it must be acknowledged as an example of paternalism.

Although respect for the autonomy of the person and his or her wishes seems central to the relationship between the client and therapist, this can sometimes be tested. Cain (p. 34), for example, quotes a situation which might apply to some of the settings in which you work. Suppose that a client whom you are seeing during their stay on a psychiatric ward tells you that she often thinks of killing herself. She also asks you not to tell the psychiatrist because she fears he will increase her medication. If you consider this a serious threat, your desire to respect the autonomy of the person will be overridden by the motive to see that no harm comes to your client. Despite the sound reasoning, this is an example of paternalism.

This discussion also shows that the professional may also need to exercise their authority to bring about change. Few therapists are in a position of possessing legal authority, except nurses in certain settings who have holding powers under the Mental Health Act. Any authority they possess will usually be founded upon their superior knowledge and the authority conferred upon them by the client. This has implications, particularly at the beginning of therapy. As Andy Farrington and Anni Telford point out in Chapter 4, the therapist must establish credibility with the client in order to gain confidence. If this display of intellectual prowess is too strong, this could compromise the goal of therapy which is to transfer knowledge and encourage self-management. However, there are times when the authority of a therapist's knowledge must be exercised and accepted by the client.

Returning to the concept of partnership, this is the characteristic that therapists would say epitomises their practice. However, partnership is a much used word in today's health and social services and warrants clarification in the context of the therapeutic relationship. First of all, partnership implies doing things **with** clients instead of **to** them. This also implies a state of equality between the client and therapist. But upon what is this equality based?

The type of equality existing between the two cannot mean equality in the literal sense of the word. It is better to see the client and therapist occupying different roles but collaborating on a joint enterprise. The therapist's role in the relationship is to make decisions concerning therapy and the client's role is to take decisions about how this can be applied to his or her lifestyle. In order to work properly, this collaboration needs to be based on a mutual respect for each other's role.

To summarise briefly, the relationship between a client and therapist is a dynamic process which can change at certain times during the therapeutic process. Overall, this relationship is one of collaboration to achieve a single objective, that being to help the client adapt to the demands of the environment. However, what qualities does the therapist need to display to make the client feel that he or she is in a collaborative relationship?

This is an aspect of therapy that has probably been the subject of more analysis than any other. Some of this research has almost obscured the need to focus equally on the more active components of therapy. In fact, the relationship itself has been seen by some to represent these active components. Lipsey and Wilson (1993), for example, showed that clients reported progress in groups in which the 'therapist' was selected for their personal positive characteristics rather than technical expertise. Caution should be expressed about such a study in that little information is given about the referring problem, which could have affected the outcome. Notwithstanding these considerations, it was Carl Rogers (1961) who highlighted the importance of the expression of interpersonal qualities, such as genuineness, warmth, empathy and acceptance of the person. These are still regarded as the key qualities of a therapist that help to develop trust and encourage collaboration. More of these qualities can be learned in the chapters that follow.

To conclude this part of the chapter, we have seen how cognitive behavioural therapy develops a self-management approach to problems. The encouragement of recent policy initiatives has not, in itself, prepared individuals to collaborate with professionals on an equal basis. Therefore, a key feature of the cognitive behavioural approach is the relationship between the client and therapist, which should be based on mutual respect and collaboration.

The professional perspective

So far, we have concentrated on factors that create needs and expectations in the individual client. It was pointed out at the beginning of this chapter that the needs and expectations of the therapist will also influence the therapeutic process. The rest of this chapter will therefore examine the context in which the professional is acquiring experience and practising therapy in order that we can make the most of our practice.

Imagine a colleague coming to you for advice. Like you, he works in a hospital. The hospital has recently restructured its management and you have now become part of a larger department with a new clinical manager. Your colleague has just come from a meeting with this manager during which he was asked to carry out more work with out-patients. The manager also told your colleague that he was concerned to target the scarce resources he had and this might involve supervising more psychology technicians in applying cognitive behavioural approaches.

Your conversation with your colleagues uncovers a few of his specific fears. 'I guess I've got used to working in one way and I'm worried about whether I'll be able to cope with the change. . . . All these questions about my job! . . . What do these technicians know anyway? . . . It's all about saving money! . . . They'll be getting people from the back of the bus queue to do our job next! . . . But what choice do I have?'

The fears expressed here represent many of the feelings that professionals have concerning the context in which they practise. These fears will inevitably create needs within the individual therapist as well as expectations about the way they should practise. The issues facing people such as the therapist above might best be summarised in terms of the following questions;

- What is the nature of professional expertise?
- How can this expertise be acquired?
- Can this expertise be transferred to different settings or groups of clients?

The following discussion will help to clarify the specific forces operating within the practice setting and will suggest ways in which these challenges can be met.

Most professionals hold beliefs that are based on expectations of a continuous improvement in their skills and a recognition by others that these skills represent a distinctive contribution. In the example given above, a threat to these beliefs is introduced. Firstly, it is suggested that non-professionals can occupy the expert position of the therapist. At the same time, however, tension is introduced by recognising the professional's skills but by suggesting that the way in which they can be recognised is through targeting these scarce resources. Essentially this tests the professional's position in relation to the view of expertise described earlier in Figure 2.4, namely, does he believe that all professional help is superior to non-professional help?

Alison Kitson (1987) examined the differences between lay and professional caring. Although this is not precisely the same as comparing these two groups in relation to therapeutic approaches, there are advantages in looking at her findings. First of all, Kitson identifies many more similarities than differences. The relationships formed with clients by lay and professional carers were characterised by trust and respect for the individual client. Motivation to care was also brought about through an emotional commitment, although the nature of this will differ between the lay and professional carer. Kitson also noticed that, whereas both groups need to recognise the limits to their own knowledge, lay caring frequently lacks the level of knowledge of the professional.

Should we be surprised or concerned about this? Also, what are the implications for the use of cognitive behavioural approaches? In the example of the therapist given earlier, this would probably provide him

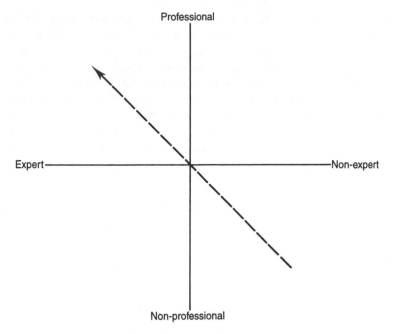

Figure 2.4   Traditional view of the hierarchy of expertise.

with some reassurance. However, in terms of the development of his practice, there are other issues he needs to acknowledge. The discrepancy in knowledge between the lay carer and the professional is an area that cognitive behaviour therapy seeks to address by giving the client the knowledge and skills eventually to act as their own therapist. However, although we would expect the client to become an expert in applying knowledge to their own problems, the therapist's knowledge is based upon the ability to enable the client to achieve this. Furthermore, it is a type of knowledge that is supported by the skills to apply therapeutic approaches to a range of clients.

Whereas this would be widely acknowledged (and the fears of the bus queue cannot be taken seriously), questions remain about the preparation of practitioners and accreditation of their practice. Anyone practising cognitive behavioural approaches in the current context of health care needs to be aware of these issues in order that clients continue to have access to such skills and that they are used to their fullest extent.

The previous decade has probably witnessed the most rapid change in the provision of health services. The impact of some of these changes is reflected in the concern of the therapist given earlier. Although these changes are numerous, the implication underpinning many of them is the need for services to clarify their responsibilities. This is essentially necessary under the new arrangements for contracting which were introduced by the NHS and Community Care Act (Department of Health 1990): services cannot be held accountable if the contract does not specify what the service is and what is the expected outcome. As far as the manager in the previous example is concerned, part of his conversation with the therapist would have been held with the objective of clarifying for him the role of the therapist in the organisation in order that decisions could then be made about the best use of his skills. It is not surprising that this creates unease.

Brown (1994) observes that the change in culture introduced in 1990 has served to destabilise many existing professional groups. Part of this destabilising effect, he claims, has been brought about by (p.60):

- The treatment of professions as trade unions.
- The questioning of long-established patterns of demarcation.
- The encouragement of local salary negotiations.
- The development of alternative qualifications to those recognised by the professions.

More recently, the National Health Service Executive (NHSE) has issued an executive letter setting out its position on alternative qualifications (NHSE 1995), saying that this is not its intention to replace existing professionals. Nevertheless, there is no doubt that the traditional working patterns of professionals have been challenged and a plethora of reviews has taken place since 1990 in order to clarify their position within the new framework for service provision (United Kingdom Chief Nursing Officers 1991; Department of Health 1994). The question is, in what way has the provision of help to individuals been affected by this change and are people in need in a better position to access appropriate help?

Professionals have long been accused of behaving in a restrictive or 'tribal' fashion. This is to say that many of them have established rituals that are unique to themselves but which may be characterised by:

- Restricting access to membership through academic qualification.
- Conducting training and education in exclusive buildings (e.g. Colleges of Nursing, Schools of Medicine).
- Controlling exit from the profession through exclusion of non-conforming members.

Other features can often include the creation of negative stereotypes of other professions, probably in order to maintain their own status and identity. This would include stereotyping non-professionals. The therapist in the example given earlier is likening the skills of the technician to those of an ordinary member of the public. Such occupational identities can be created within a few months of a person entering professional training (Pietroni 1991). On the other hand, whereas professions may possess these characteristics, many professionals themselves emphasise the positive aspects of professionalism, such as being a source of expertise, taking ownership of a particular problem or need, and being decisive and accountable for their practice. For this reason, professions enjoy a high status within society and the trust of the majority of the public.

Some of the negative aspects of professionalism have been addressed in recent times, especially since the health service reforms. Together with the need for clarity, collaboration between services and professions has been an essential feature of much of the guidance from the Department of Health. Amongst other things, it is hoped that this will enable a greater focus upon need and create better understanding of the contribution of different professionals. Furthermore, the education of some professionals has been relocated to sites in which contact with other groups is more likely to happen.

However, expectations of professionals concerning their own practice can adversely affect the degree of access of the public to this expertise. For example, some professionals, such as psychologists and psychiatrists have traditionally worked in hospital settings. If the beliefs of people such as this are that these are the only places in which therapy can be applied, the potential benefits of therapy will not be realised. Furthermore, anyone wishing to learn about and acquire such skills would have similar problems of access. Would we advise the therapist in the earlier example to work towards the changes required by his manager?

The solution to this simple scenario might seem perfectly obvious to us but issues such as these have raised huge questions concerning the transportability and transferability of special skills. In this sense, transportability refers to the different settings in which help can be provided. For example, open heart surgery is not an easily transportable form of treatment. Transferability refers to the extent to which skills can be acquired by a range of people as well as the range of problems these skills can address. For example, can people without qualifications in clinical psychology provide help for people with depression and can these skills also be used to help someone with an obsessive–compulsive disorder?

In 1986, the Department of Employment and the Department of Education and Science (DoE and DES 1986) published a document, which outlined the need to make education and training more relevant to improving the skills and competence of the workforce in order to create jobs, open new career opportunities and create wealth. The essential features of the approach that developed from this document was one in which competence can be assessed against a set of criteria, or occupational standards, which are determined by the needs of the particular job. A system of National Vocational Qualifications (NVQs) was therefore developed, which could be applied to a wide range of occupations.

Jessup (1991) describes this development in more detail. However, in the area of caring for people, the Care Sector Consortium introduced NVQs for a range of staff who previously would have had little or no access to formal qualifications. The professional response to this development has been mixed. However, in almost every area of professional training, courses are now modularised with 'credits' awarded to the individuals undertaking them. These modules, or credits, can be accumulated and transferred to obtain qualifications. Clifton (1994) explains this process in more detail, but the intention is to create a system of national standards for education and training similar to that of the Care Sector Consortium.

Despite the apparent competition between these approaches, it should not be regarded as a threat to professionalism. Competence-based training is a challenge to incompetence, not to expertise. Waitman (1992) makes the point that, in the desire to make skills accessible to a wider range of people in the past, the result has been an increase in short courses, for example, in counselling, which have served only to encourage the 'amateur with talent'. Waitman rightly argues that this has devalued the person needing help and the status of therapeutic approaches, such as cognitive behaviour therapy. The current emphasis on competence presents an opportunity to reverse this process. This is a move which is wholly endorsed by the contributors to this book. Furthermore, all of the contributors believe not only that many people can acquire competencies in therapeutic approaches but that many of them are already demonstrating their competence in these areas.

In terms of our disgruntled therapist, this might help convince him of the need to accept change. The technician clearly offers no threat if both of them are prepared to develop their practice according to clear competencies that are defined by the needs of the job.

Conclusion

This chapter opened by using a diagram to describe how the therapeutic encounter between the client and therapist is just one aspect of a larger process. Prior to entering therapy, both client and therapist will have experiences that shape the way they think. Ultimately this will affect the way they view themselves and their approach to therapy. As far as the client is concerned, these beliefs may include expectations of cure or of playing a passive role in therapy. The client therefore requires greater clarification of the situations that give rise to needs, and the role he or she must play in meeting them. The therapist needs to acknowledge that the context in which he or she is practising is one that is moving towards increased clarification of the skills needed to meet the needs of clients. Therefore, although each person's needs are distinctive, they are mutually beneficial.

Discussion questions

1. From where does the public get its information about therapy? How could this image be improved?
2. The Health of the Nation policy sets out targets for mental health. What role could be played by cognitive behaviour therapy in achieving these targets?
3. Would you describe a competent therapist as a specialist or advanced nursing practitioner?

References

Barker, P. (1989) Reflections on the philosophy of caring in mental health. **International Journal of Nursing Studies** 26, 131–141.
Brown, J. (1994) **The Hybrid Worker.** York: University of York, Department of Social Policy and Social Work.
Cain, P. (1995) Community nurse–client relations. In Cain, P., Hyde, V. and Howkins, L. (eds) **Community Nursing: Dimensions and Dilemmas.** London: Edward Arnold. pp. 27–41.
Clifton, M. (1994) **Training and Education in transition: bridging vocational and academic models in an interdisciplinary perspective.** York: University of York, Department of Social Policy and Social Work.
Department of Employment and Department of Education and Science (1986) **Working Together – Education and Training.** London: HMSO.
Department of Health (1990) **NHS and Community Care Act.** London: HMSO.
Department of Health (1991) **The Patients' Charter.** London: HMSO.
Department of Health (1992) **The Health of the Nation: A Strategy for Health in England.** London: HMSO.
Department of Health (1994) **Working in Partnership: A Collaborative Approach to Care.** Report of the Mental Health Nursing Review Team. London: Department of Health.
Horvath, A.O. and Greenberg, L.S. (1993) **The Working Alliance: Theory, Research and Practice.** New York: Wiley.

Jessup, G. (1991) **Outcomes: The Emerging Model of Education and Training.** London: Falmer Press.

Kahn, J. and Earle, E. (1982) **The Cry for Help and the Professional Response.** Oxford: Pergammon Press.

Kitson, A.L. (1987) A comparative analysis of lay caring and professional (nursing) caring relationships. **International Journal of Nursing Studies** 24, 155–165.

Lipsey, M.W. and Wilson, D.B. (1993) The efficacy of psychological, educational and behavioural treatment. **American Psychologist** December, 1181–2009.

National Health Service Executive (1995) **Building on the Benefits of Occupational Standards and National Vocational Qualifications (NVQs) in the NHS.** EL(95)84. London: National Health Service Executive.

Pietroni, P.C. (1991) Stereotypes or archetypes – a study of perceptions among health care students. **Journal of Social Work Practice** 5, 61–69.

Rogers, C. (1961) **On Becoming a Person.** London: Constable.

United Kingdom Chief Nursing Officers (1991) **Mental Handicap Nursing in the Context of 'Caring for People'.** London: Department of Health.

Waitman, A. (1992) Demystifying traditional approaches to counselling and psychotherapy. In Waitman A. and Conboy-Hill S. (eds) **Psychotherapy and Mental Handicap.** London: Sage, pp. 202–220.

Further reading

Cain, P. (1995) The ethical dimension. In Cain P., Hyde V. and Howkins E. **Community Nursing: Dimensions and Dilemmas.** London: Edward Arnold.

Priestly, P. and McGuire, J. (1983) **Learning to help. Basic skills exercises.** London: Tavistock Publications.

United Kingdom Central Council (1994) **The future of professional practice – the Council's standards for education and practice following registration.** London: UKCC.

Wilson-Barnett, J. (1989) Limited autonomy and partnership: professional relations in health care. **Journal of Medical Ethics.** 15: 12–16.

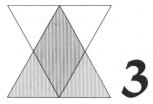

3

The Characteristics of Cognitive Behaviour Therapy

Sue Marshall

Key issues

- Core characteristics of cognitive behaviour therapy
- Theoretical origins of cognitive behaviour therapy
- Links between cognitive behaviour therapy and nursing practice competencies

---

Overview

This chapter is divided into three parts. In the first part there is a brief introduction to those characteristics that we propose as central or core themes in the practice of cognitive behaviour therapy. This includes a brief review of some of the work carried out by psychologists who developed theories that have been influential in moulding the way cognitive behaviour therapy is practised today. This is followed by a detailed description of each of these characteristics. Next comes an account of how aspects of nursing practice reflect elements of the characteristics described.

One view of cognitive behaviour therapy _____

This book takes a particular view about the central themes of cognitive behaviour therapy. We suggest that there are four core characteristics of cognitive behaviour therapy that are influential in terms of outcome. Irrespective of the specific nature of the persons presenting problems, we consider these characteristics to be fundamental. These characteristics are:

- The nature of the therapeutic relationship.
- The use of strategies that aim to identify and rectify dysfunctional cognitions.
- Maximising success and opportunities by planning for times when things do not go according to plan.
- Ensuring that all aspects of the therapeutic encounter are the subject of clinical supervision.

Other texts identify other features, and highlight different aspects or elements of the therapy as being central to it (Dryden and Golden 1986). Fundamental to all work in the area is a common belief in the influential nature of cognitions on behaviour (Robins and Hayes 1993). Irrespective of what else may be identified as important in any particular brand of this therapy, this basic assumption is fundamental to the practice of cognitive behaviour therapy. What follows is one particular expression of how that basic assumption can be put into practice.

In the following chapter, these core characteristics are presented as themes, which can be identified throughout the various stages of the therapy process: the process that you go through with a client who is referred for therapy, starting with assessment and ending in discharge.

Moving from assessment to maintenance: the sequence of a therapeutic encounter

Below is a very brief overview of the stages involved in the therapeutic process. In the next three chapters of the book this process is expanded upon and the detail of how you move from assessment to maintenance is described.

Throughout the time you work with a client it is important to recognize the limits of your competence and work within this limit. Supervision helps to ensure that you are practising within the limits of your competence.

As with any therapeutic intervention, the first step must be to define the difficulties the person is having. This assessment informs the formulation of the problem and helps to identify outcomes or aims for therapy. The unique element of assessment in cognitive behaviour therapy is to identify links between thoughts, feelings and behaviour. To do this, you must work on current events. You will ask the client to describe what is happening in their life, what are the things that are difficult for them, what are the things they feel are satisfactory. In addition to current events, you will need to ask about their personal history. You may use a standardised self-report checklist to help elicit information. These are commercially available assessments which have been designed to assist in the assessment process.

A standardised assessment is one that has been developed and tested with a large number of people. The results for all these people are gathered together. Those questions that are consistently answered in a particular way are kept in the assessment. Those questions that are answered in a variety of different ways are removed from the final list of questions. These questions are removed because they are not predictive. That is, the answer to the questions do not help to predict if a person is depressed or anxious, for example, in comparison to the rest of the population.

In completing an assessment, you will ask the client to do a homework task. This will often include asking the person to keep a diary of the week's events. You will need to specify exactly what they should record. It is important that the client is clear about what you are asking of them. In doing this you should be sensitive to any concerns the person may have, however trivial they may appear to be. The skilled and sensitive therapist will ensure that the person thinks they are able to participate fully in the task. More detailed descriptions of diary keeping can be found in Chapter 4.

It is particularly important that in this early stage of the relationship you make the client feel secure and valued. They must not be put in a position where they see themselves in danger of failing in any way. Homework tasks should be achievable for the client.

To ensure this is the case, you may have to adapt tried and tested methods of enabling the client to complete their homework. For example, if the person is not a native English speaker, or they have difficulties with reading and writing, it is no good asking them to keep a written diary.

Once the assessment phase is completed, then the intervention stage can begin. You will have a whole array of techniques that you can employ to assist the client in altering the way they think about the various problems that face them. These are described briefly below and in more detail in Chapter 5.

As time goes on and the client makes progress, so the process moves into a generalisation and maintenance phase as described in Chapter 6. This is when the client takes on increasingly more responsibility for their self-management and, in collaboration with you, they direct the therapy. In order to do this the person will have to spend time planning how they intend to maximise successes and opportunities, and how they will minimise the effect of barriers that will be presented to them. They are

Table 3.1 The sequence of an episode of therapy

	Assessment and formulation (Chapter 4)	Intervention (Chapter 5)	Generalisation and maintenance (Chapter 6)
Relationships	*	*	*
Strategies	*	*	*
When things do not go as planned	*	*	*
Supervision	*	*	*

planning for when things do not go to plan. To prepare them, you should have modelled this throughout the therapeutic process for the client, employing a range of skills to ensure that the person is realistic about their situation (see Table 3.1).

What is the aim of cognitive therapy?

Adaptation is the process whereby an individual changes to suit a new set of conditions or circumstances. When a person is in good health, they behave adaptively. They respond to changes in a way that enables them to continue to function in the altered environment.

The aim of cognitive behaviour therapy is to allow the person to take control of his or her own problems and for him or her to manage his/her life in such a way that future problems are dealt with in an adaptive way. Mahoney (1993) has described this as the cognitive therapies' 'commitment to self-examination and self-awareness'.

As previously described, cognitive behaviour therapy is useful not only for people with mental health problems. A look at the contents of a book about the practice of the therapy will illustrate the range of difficulties with which it is used (Dryden and Rentoul 1991), this includes helping people to cope with physical health problems, relationship difficulties, pain management, stress management and the development of social skills. In all of these areas the aim is the same, that is, for the person to manage their lives adaptively by recognising the interaction between thoughts, feelings and behaviour.

During therapy the amount of control individuals accept for themselves will vary. One aim should be that, by the time the person is discharged, the therapist has minimal control and the client is able to cope with his or her difficulties. This is achieved by the client recognising the relationship between thoughts, feelings and behaviour. In this way they will be able to influence the way they feel, by altering the way they think about events.

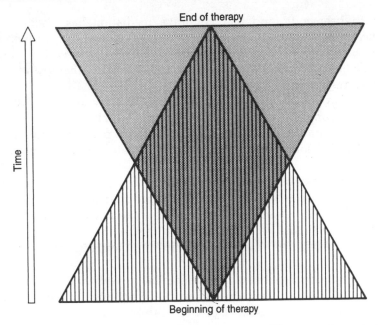

Figure 3.1 The emergence of self-management. ⬚, proportion of therapy directed by the therapist; ▨, proportion of therapy directed by the client.

This is not to say that they will never need help in the future. However, they should be able to minimise the negative effects of future difficult life events.

The process of recognition, and the transfer of management and skills from the therapist to the client is illustrated above (Figure 3.1).

Clearly progression for individuals in therapy will vary, but the general theme will persist. Initially, the therapist, in collaboration with the client, directs the course of therapy. As time goes on, the client, in collaboration with the therapist, directs the therapy. At the point of discharge, the therapist should have handed over control to the client. They should be able to manage their lives in such a way as to minimise the effects of any future problems. The client should now be able to recognise clearly and manipulate the complex relationship between thoughts, feelings and behaviour.

What are the basic assumptions made by cognitive behaviour therapists?

There are a number of basic assumptions made by cognitive behaviour therapists. These are that cognitions are real; that cognitions are the medium via which behaviour is prompted, that is they act as mediating factors in behaviour; and that cognitive mediation has a significant influence on a person's behaviour. For you, as a therapist, to help the client to achieve this understanding, you should have a sound knowledge of the theoretical background of cognitive behaviour therapy and the basic assumptions of the model.

The term 'cognition' is used in psychology to refer to many different things, for example, it can be used to mean ideas, attributions, expectations, conceptions, meaning. 'Cognitions' form part of many major psychological theories, even some which predate cognitive behaviour therapy.

As already described in Chapter 2, cognitive behaviour therapy is a collection of varied techniques that can be grouped together under one broad heading. However, cognitive behaviour therapy is not an arbitrary collection of tools and techniques. It is a therapy based on a unifying philosophy about the interrelationship of thoughts, feelings and behaviour.

Some of the techniques used may be familiar to you, for example, many of them are used in behavioural work. What marks the cognitive behaviour therapist out is a set of basic assumptions about the central nature of cognitions. Many of the techniques, as I have suggested, are used elsewhere but their successful application within the cognitive behavioural framework will only be achieved if the role of cognitions is always recognised as crucial.

Some important theoretical influences by 'non-cognitivists'

Kelly (1955): Personal construct theory

Kelly developed 'personal construct theory' in which he described people as scientists who interpret the events that go on around them (Kelly 1955). These interpretations are based on personal templates. These are like blueprints that individuals develop through their experience of the world. These templates Kelly called personal constructs.

Everyone builds up their own personal constructs, which they use to impose meaning on events in their world. People do this in an effort to make their world predictable.

Kelly proposed that individuals use their personal construct to anticipate the outcome of events. If the prediction matches the outcome of events, then the personal construct is validated. The validity of the construct may be called into question by the individual if the outcome of events does not match their prediction. The person can then go on to alter their personal construct using the results of their latest experience.

When the person does not alter the construct in light of their experience, the result will be confusion and an inability to make sense of their world. According to Kelly, psychological distress results from an inability to revise constructs.

Although he predates the development of cognitive behaviour therapy, Kelly's theory illustrates the importance of cognitions in identifying and working with psychological distress.

It is easy to imagine how this theory would work in practice. Consider the person who, because of past experience develops a personal construct, which suggests that they do not like going to parties where there is a large crowd. This will influence the way they look forward to going to a party. The result of this anticipation is likely to be an increase in stress, which in turn may influence their ability to relax and enjoy the party. What if, despite their expectations, they do enjoy the party? They can use this experience to influence and adapt their personal construct about parties. If they are unable to do this, their construct about parties will remain unchallenged, so the next time they are invited out the chances are that they will be distressed at the prospect.

The important point to recognise from Kelly's work is the role of expectation and anticipation in helping us to make sense of the world.

Although his theory predates most work done in the development of cognitive behaviour therapy, it demonstrates that cognitions in one guise or another have been a feature of psychological theory for some time and that their influential role on behaviour has long been recognised.

Tolman (1932): Mediational model of behaviour

It was Tolman (1932) who first introduced the idea that an internal process occurs between an observable stimulus event and an observable response to that event. He argued that, between an event and a response, there is some kind of internal representation of the event. Tolman suggested that this helps the individual to make some kind of judgement about how best to respond to what is going on around them.

His ideas came from his observations of the behaviour of rats in a maze. Tolman demonstrated that rats would find the shortest route through a maze if they could obtain some reinforcement at the end of their search. The rats would vary their route to find the quickest way to the reinforcement.

Tolman argued that people, like rats, use internal representations of events to help them solve problems in their environment. On the basis of his experimental work, he proposed that the relationship between an event and a response is not straightforward. The response depends on some intervening mental event, what cognitive behaviour therapists call a cognition. Tolman's view of behaviour became known as the mediational model of behaviour.

Bandura (1977): Social learning theory

Bandura (1977) extended Tolman's mediational model of behaviour in his description of social learning theory.

Social learning theorists like Bandura emphasise that individual patterns of behaviour develop because of an interaction between the person and their environment. Patterns of behaviour can be acquired either through direct experience or by observing the behaviour of other people.

Cognitive processes are stressed in a way that is similar to Tolman's and to Kelly's theory of behaviour. The social learning theorist recognise that people can represent situations symbolically in their heads. This allows us to anticipate the possible outcome of events and to decide on a course of action.

The action we take may be the result of a previous similar experience, or it may be the result of our observations of other people in similar situations. We usually adopt a course that will have a positive outcome for us. In doing this we ascribe a value to that outcome. Behaviour which provides us with a desired outcome is reinforced and is likely to be displayed again. Behaviour which does not provide us with what we want is unlikely to be displayed again.

Rotter (1975): Reinforcement value

Rotter called this 'reinforcement value' (Rotter and Hochreich 1975). If a person ascribes a high value to the reinforcement they obtain from behaving in a particular way, the probability of this behaviour being repeated in similar circumstances is high. In ascribing this value, our behaviour is influenced by cognitions. If someone ascribes a low value to the reinforcement they obtain for behaving in a particular way, the likelihood of this behaviour being repeated in similar circumstances is low.

An everyday example of this would be a student who is awarded a 'C' after working particularly hard on an essay. If the student usually gets 'C', then it is unlikely that they will consider the extra effort worth the mark awarded. Their changed behaviour has not been reinforced by the response it received and the chance of it occurring again is not increased by the reinforcement offered. If, however, the student usually gets a 'D' and they consider the increased effort worth making, their changed behaviour will be influenced by the reinforcement they ascribe to their better mark. The person has made a judgement about relative value of the reinforcement.

Yet, even in this simple example, the complexity of the relationship between how we think and how we behave is apparent. Consider all the potential variables in the apparently simple scenario above. The value of the reinforcement may be influenced by the person who is responsible for awarding the mark. It could be affected by the subject of the essay, or the relative value of the mark achieved, if the person compares their mark with those of their peers. These are just a few of the variables that could influence the perceived value of the reinforcement.

An array of factors come into play when considering the reinforcement value individuals ascribe to events. This simple example above highlights the complexity of human behaviour, and begins to illustrate the potential flaws in describing behaviour in terms of a simple linear relationship between a stimulus and a response (Pavlov 1927) without considering the intervening role of cognitions.

None of the theorists described above would describe themselves as cognitive behaviour therapist, but all have had an important role to play in the development of cognitive behaviour therapy. In the seminal works of Beck (1976), Ellis (1962) and Meichenbaum (1977), the influence of theories described above is clear.

The constructivist view

Cognitive behaviour therapists have a constructivist view of people. This means that individuals are considered to be active in the way they think about their world. People are viewed as complex systems in which thoughts, feelings and behaviour are interdependent.

The elements of the system develop during people's lives as they interact with the social system in which they live. The product of this development is the construction of a set of schema (Beck and Emery 1985). Schema are similar to Kelly's constructs described above. They direct how people interpret what is going on around them and inform how they think about events. Cognitive behaviour therapy proposes that thoughts, feelings and behaviour are inextricably linked. It follows therefore that identification of schema with the client is a crucial outcome of cognitive behaviour therapy.

The seminal theorists in cognitive behaviour therapy have different approaches to their practice of the therapy. The language they use to describe their practice is also diverse. Despite this diversity, therapists practising cognitive behaviour therapy always have a constructivist view of individuals. The philosophical basis for the therapy is this shared view of the influential role of thoughts in the expression of affect (feelings) and the display of behaviour.

An example of the constructivist approach might be the work of Arron Beck. Beck's cognitive behaviour theory of the origins and maintaining factors in depression identifies a 'negative cognitive triad'. This triad is composed of a schema in which the person holds a negative view of themselves, of the world and of the future. The triad arises from the interaction between real experiences and the individual's attempts to impose a meaning on those events. Ultimately the results of this interaction becomes a part of the person's long-term memory and operates as a schema for the person (Beck 1967).

The schema is accessible through the overt expression of automatic thoughts and influences a person's mood and their behaviour (see Figure 3.2). Automatic thoughts are the thoughts which spring into your mind apparently from nowhere. They are not those produced by sitting down and thinking through a problem. Schema can be identified via automatic thoughts of the person. They often seem to the individual to be arbitrary and unrelated, but they reflect the basic assumptions or beliefs contained within a schema that a person holds.

Ellis's model of depression places an emphasis on the basic beliefs or assumptions the person holds (see Figure 3.2). What Beck calls schema, Ellis calls beliefs. It is beliefs that give rise to the tendency for a person to evaluate events in a way that results in depressed feelings. These evaluations can be recognised by the way the person talks about an event and their tendency to use dogmatic terms such as 'must', 'have to' and 'should do'. The person's belief system is sparked off by an event; in responding to their belief system the person sets exacting standards for themselves. The standards may be so high and inflexible that they do not fulfil these expectations. The result is they feel inadequate and depressed.

Figure 3.2 illustrates how the major theorists in cognitive behaviour therapy use different terms to reflect their individual perspectives in theory. Beck describes schema, Ellis writes of beliefs and Meichenbaum uses concepts to describe the underlying structures that affect the way we think (our cognitions) about events that happen (Ellis 1962, Meichenbaum 1977).

All these exponents of cognitive behaviour therapy maintain that underlying structures are influential for the client and are accessible. Access can be achieved via reporting of self-statements and automatic thoughts. These then become the focus of attention during therapy. The fundamental task of therapy is to alter schema and thereby influence how the person feels.

When the automatic thoughts have a negative effect on the way the person thinks and feels, they are described as dysfunctional cognitions. During therapy you will use a range of techniques to alter these dysfunctional cognitions. By doing this, you are working to affect the underlying structures by influencing the more accessible structures. This is illustrated in Figure 3.2.

Having described some of the theoretical background to cognitive behaviour therapy, I want to return to the four core characteristics

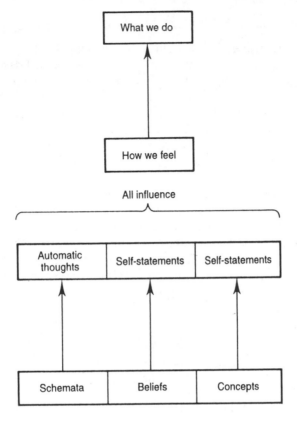

Figure 3.2   The relationship between thoughts, feelings and behaviour.

introduced at the beginning of the chapter. Each of these will be referred to in subsequent chapters describing how they are addressed at various stages of the therapeutic process.

The therapeutic relationship

When working with a client and using cognitive behaviour therapy, the nature of the relationship between the client and you, as the therapist, is crucial. Rogers has described the ideal therapeutic relationship as being characterised by its warmth, the genuineness of the relationship and unconditional positive regard shown by the therapist to the client (Rogers 1967). Warmth is defined by the accuracy of the empathy expressed by the therapist.

Accuracy

Accuracy can be judged by the fit between the way the therapist describes a client's problem and the way the client himself or herself describes his or her problem. For a good fit the therapist needs to make an accurate assessment, taking full account of the client's perspective of the problem. In arriving at a definition or formulation of the problem, you, the therapist, will reinterpret and reframe the client's problem. This is best done in a way that allows your client to recognise that you are describing his or her problem, not something which has little personal significance for the client.

When you describe your client's problem, you should use the same language that the client has used when he or she described it initially. This is especially important when reflecting back how the problem makes the person feel – if the person says he or she feels lousy, then that is what the person means, and you should try to use the same adjective he or she has used. It is, of course, legitimate to ask for clarification of a particular word or expression, so it may be that you ask 'What do you mean by lousy? Tell me a bit more about that'.

In seeking clarification about feelings, it is important not to challenge the person aggressively. Instead foster a feeling of collaboration with the client so that he or she thinks you have a genuine interest in finding out as much as you can about his or her problem, so that you can offer the client the help he or she is asking for.

As the therapist, you may think differently from the client about what is keeping the problem going. However, you must take the client's word about how the problem is making him or her feel. You should assume that the client's view of his or her problems is internally consistent. It may not be technically correct or logical. It may be idiosyncratic, but it will be consistent. Recognising this and using it as you work will help to establish a warm relationship that the client thinks of as secure and positive. One in which the client's problems are taken account of accurately.

Accuracy will also be demonstrated if you ask for feedback and clarification. If, for example, the client has described something to you about the effect his or her problem has on his or her life and it is not clear to you what they mean, it is important to make sure you check your understanding with the client. In doing this you should take responsibility for the fact that you are not sure about what the client means. The client should not be left thinking that it is their fault that you are unclear.

It is during the early stages of therapy that the client develops a schema that will inform the way they feel about both the therapist and therapy. It is critical that this schema give rise to positive thoughts and feelings about the relationship that he or she is developing with the therapist. In seeking feedback, you are helping to establish this positive relationship, defined by trust and a sense of collaboration between yourself and the client.

During the whole episode of therapy, the client's response to you will be informed by this schema he or she has developed. Thinking of you in a positive way as someone who understands his or her difficulties and has the skills to help him or her will establish a good working relationship. The client is more likely, therefore to accept your reframing of his or her problems and to participate in tasks you set him or her.

You may confront resistance during therapy. At this early assessment stage, this may reflect a general schema about significant people in the client's life. It is important that the client thinks of you as different from other people in his or her life – particularly those who may have, unsuccessfully, tried to help them. The person has come for therapy because, for some reason, their ordinary supports and networks have not been perceived by them as helpful with the problems they are now experiencing. It is highly likely that the person is coming for therapy only after he or she has tried a whole range of other things. Through this the person will have developed a collection of expectations about the outcome of well-intentioned help. These expectations will collectively form a schema, which will be influential in how the person thinks and feels about your help.

You may have to work hard to distance yourself from this pre-existing schema and to offer the client some new evidence to challenge it. By establishing yourself as a therapist with whom he or she can have a relationship, which is characterised by a genuine understanding of his or her problem, the client will be encouraged to participate in the therapeutic process and to develop a positive schema about therapeutic relationships.

Supervision offers the opportunity to reflect on the way the client thinks about you. This can be a useful place to consider not only the schema the client may be developing about you, but how you think about the client.

After the assessment phase is complete, the client should think that you have an accurate understanding of his or her problem. This accuracy should be reflected when you negotiate goals and outcomes for therapy. These goals should be shared and should accurately summarise the aims of the client seeking help. They should also be realistic.

Genuineness

The second aspect of therapeutic relationships identified by Rogers is that of 'genuineness'. Genuineness is the ability of the therapist to express to the client the various thoughts and feelings they have about the relationship. It can be tested at points during the relationship. Your client may have a particular goal in mind, which you recognise to be unobtainable or which may be self-defeating. When this happens, you have a responsibility to make your thoughts and feelings clear to the client.

Genuineness is directly related to unconditional positive regard. Within the context of person-centred psychotherapy, unconditional positive regard is described as a willingness to care for the client irrespective of the way the client is behaving (Rogers 1967). Rogers describes the therapist as having always to think of the client in an unreservedly positive way. This can be misconstrued by the therapist, who adopts a passive and unquestioning role in their relationship with the client. In cognitive behaviour therapy this may lead to a situation where no change is possible because the therapist is not able to challenge their client.

There is a difference between such passivity and an active, sometimes directive genuineness that results in opportunities for the client to change. Within a cognitive behavioural framework, there are risks in offering unconditional positive regard, if it results in a non-directive approach when people act out their difficulties. When a client displays behaviour, or reports thoughts and feelings that are unhelpful, you should actively encourage the client to consider the implications of their thoughts and behaviour. Take, for example, a client who says that they think that the homework that you have set them will not help them to gain any additional insight into their thoughts or feelings. They say they have a right not to participate in tasks that they think are meaningless. If you passively agree that the client can opt out of this aspect of the therapy, you lose a valuable opportunity to encourage the client to think about what their automatic thoughts are about this particular situation. You can use such live pieces of data to help in the cognitive restructuring and formulation of the client's problem.

A note of caution

By now I hope that the role of cognitions in cognitive behaviour therapy is becoming clearer. The defining philosophy of the therapy is based on the idea that cognitive distortions in our basic assumptions give rise to negative schema, which in some circumstances create emotional distress. This distress arises from the influence of schema giving rise to automatic thoughts that have a negative influence on the person's feelings and their behaviour. The link between thoughts, feelings and behaviour is a fundamental issue in cognitive behaviour therapy.

It follows, therefore, that all the strategies used by a cognitive behaviour therapist aim to influence feelings and behaviour by effecting some change in the way the person thinks about what is going on in their world. Such practice has obvious ethical implications, these are discussed in detail in Chapter 7 and, before you embark on therapy, it is a good idea to spend time thinking about the ethics of what you are about to do. After thinking about the ethical implications of cognitive behaviour therapy, review your understanding of the underlying philosophy of the therapy.

Cognitive behaviour therapy sometimes seems to lend itself to a cookbook approach to working with people. There are, however, a number of workers who warn against the dangers of this apparent eclecticism and tolerance for a range of techniques. They are critical of texts that describe the 'tools of the trade' and do not ensure that the fundamental principles of the therapy are given due attention (Gilbert 1993). The reader should be familiar with this literature before they embark upon any therapy. The arguments rehearsed in it represent an important strand of knowledge. Without a recognition of the unifying principles of cognitive behaviour, therapy tools and techniques will be used without insight. This may result in 'treatment failures'.

Strategies for restructuring cognitive dysfunction

Cognitive restructuring is at the heart of cognitive behaviour therapy. According to Beck there are a number of ways in which a person's thinking can become dysfunctional. Below is a brief description of some of the ways in which thinking can become distorted. Collectively these distortions are called 'cognitive dysfunctions'.

Black and white thinking is where a person cannot discriminate between a range of possible alternative interpretations of an event. Rather they interpret events as either wholly positive or wholly negative. There are no grey areas in this person's view of the world. An example of the expression of black and white thinking is when you hear someone describe a situation as completely hopeless. When, in reality, there are some positive features to it.

A student who gains a 'B' grade for an assignment, where the class average is a 'C', and describes his or her performance as 'useless' would be thinking in black and white terms. This would be particularly true if the student's previous average grade was an 'A'. In such a case the person would not be looking at all the evidence available to him or her.

The same person may think that a peer who scored a 'C' had done perfectly well, but will not accept that they should be judged by the same criteria. In this case they would be applying a different set of rules to judge their own behaviour in comparison to another student's.

Typical of the person whose cognitions are dysfunctional is the tendency to use 'should' and 'must' when talking about their expectations of himself/herself. Such a way of thinking increases the demands that individuals place on themselves with the result that they are constantly dissatisfied with their performance.

The person who engages in cognitive distortions will often reject all the positive aspects of a particular event. Going back to the student who is awarded a grade 'B' when the class average is a 'C'. They will not think 'it's not as high as my usual mark, but it is still above average – this must have been a very difficult piece of work'. They will miss out all of the qualifying parts of the sentence and not consider the reasons or evidence for their mark being different from previous performances. The emotional affect caused is one of disappointment and dissatisfaction with themselves.

Catastrophising is another example of a common cognitive distortion. Elaborating the example above of the student; if they say that their performance on this assignment indicates that they will never again be able to get a grade 'A', they are catastrophising. They take one episode and judge their future by it. In addition, they will fail to take account of past experiences or minimise previous events, which may contradict this recent evidence. They maximise the meaning of this latest piece of evidence.

This student is constantly monitoring his or her environment and, because of the way s/he interprets and anticipates events, s/he will find evidence to support his or her dysfunctional view of the world and their place in it. If you were the student's therapist, your task would be to help him or her to recognise that the way s/he thinks about events is having an effect on the way s/he feels. Then, to help the student alter the way s/he thinks and to use a more constructive or adaptive way of thinking.

This then is the task of cognitive behaviour therapy. The chapters which follow will offer a range of strategies to help you, as a therapist, to bring this about. What follows below is a brief introduction to these strategies.

The purpose of cognitive restructuring is to make the client reconsider how they view the world and to begin to consider that there may be another way of thinking about things. This should be done during a therapy session with the client using material they bring to the session. This will often be in the form of a diary, which the client will be asked to keep. During these sessions, as a therapist, you will model various methods designed to help the client re-evaluate their view. You will ask the client to analyse his or her interpretation of events. A good way of doing this is to use questions that are thought provoking. If someone comes to see you because they think they cannot get on with people in a social situation, the session may proceed like that described below.

Client: I cannot go to the party that I have been invited to because I will not enjoy it.

Therapist: Are you confusing thoughts with facts? How can you be so sure that you will not enjoy yourself?

Client: Well, OK. I don't know that I won't enjoy it but what if the only other people that are there are people who do not know me?

Therapist: Are you predicting the future? How do you know that there will not be anyone there who knows you?

Client: Even if I do know them, I bet they will all be in couples and won't want to be bothered talking to me.

Therapist: Are you thinking in black and white terms here? Do you know for sure that any of your concerns will be borne out by the facts?

The discussion would proceed with you trying gradually to encourage your client to think about the event differently. The aim is have the client agree to go to the party and to test out their fears.

In preparing the client to go to the party, it is important for you to set very clear goals with him or her. The objective is for the client to do some reality testing. Reality testing is about gathering evidence to discount specific thoughts the client has that impact on their difficulties. You may agree, for example, that they could go to the party to check if everyone else is in couples. Even if this turns out to be the case, does it naturally follow that no one wants to speak to them? Evidence collected at the party can then be used to challenge the client's negative assumptions – his or her basic view of him/herself. In this way, they can reframe and change what they think and therefore fear about similar future events.

Reframing is a way of offering a markedly different interpretation of events. It is often an opposite interpretation. In the example given above, where you have agreed with the client that they will go to the party to check their assumption that everyone will be in couples and that no one will make any effort to speak to them, it may be that in the next session they will report the evening to have been a disaster. The discussion may proceed something like this:

Therapist: How did you get on at the party? Were you able to get the information we agreed you would try to get?

Client: Well, yes, I did, but the evening was a disaster, I had a terrible time!

Therapist: What do you mean by a disaster?

Client: Nearly every one was in a couple and I felt like they were only interested in each other.

Therapist: Not everyone was in a couple then?

Client: No, not everyone was. But at least half of the people there were in a couple.

Therapist: So about how many of the people there were unattached?

Client: About half, I guess.

Therapist: Rather than the evening being a disaster could you think of it as a success? You were able to check out your assumption that everyone would be part of a couple and that you would be the odd one out. It seems from what you have said, that in fact only half of the people there were part of a couple. Do you think you could use this information next time you are invited out? Do you think it would help you to feel less anxious if you used this evidence that you have gathered?

By reframing this experience with the client, you are modelling how to use real evidence and how to avoid overgeneralisation when reviewing the results of an event. It would be easy for you to get caught up with the client's general feeling that everything had gone wrong. However, by setting clear goals that focus on aspects of an experience that is influenced by cognitive distortions, a positive outcome is likely. This allows the client to start to gain real-life examples, which will provide a corrective to assumptions based on cognitive distortions.

Problem solving is another useful tool to help the person to consider alternative interpretations of events. The process of problem solving involves the client thinking through the answers to several questions. The questions are:

- What is the problem?
- What are the possible solutions?
- Which is the solution that best helps me?

Once the client has arrived at their solution, then they should put their solution into practice and evaluate the outcome.

The solutions are derived from a process of brainstorming, which you guide the client through. The crucial thing about brainstorming is that any potential solution should be recorded, however unusual it is. It is only after the brainstorming that the client evaluates the options and chooses the one which s/he thinks would be the most helpful. Then negotiate with the client about trying to use this alternative interpretation of events when next they are presented with a similar situation. By doing this the client will be attempting to do things differently and to gather evidence that they can use to reframe the way they think about such events in the future.

When a client is able to make any change in their behaviour, you should encourage them to reinforce themselves for making that change.

Self-reinforcement is another essential tool for you to pass on to the client. Reinforcement is the term used to describe something that has the effect of strengthening a bond of association, which has developed between two events – a stimulus and a response. Self-reinforcement is especially important when the client has been discharged from therapy; self-reinforcement helps the client to be their own therapist. Studies have shown that, for people who are taught to use self-reinforcement, the chances of generalisation and maintenance of a newly acquired skill is increased (Whitman et al. 1987; Marshall 1992). Clients who use self-reinforcement do not rely on an external control (usually the therapist) for feedback. Meichenbaum refers to this as self-inoculation and it is a prominent feature of many anxiety- and anger-management strategies.

Supervision and reflective practice

A recent position paper prepared for the Department of Health (Faugier and Butterworth 1993), identified the need for supervision to become a central feature of nursing practice, across all of its branches. The paper highlights the difference between clinical supervision and managerial supervision. It emphasises the need to ensure that practitioners have access to a range of expertise to support them during their clinical practice. The paper offers a range of definitions of supervision and identifies Wright's definition as being the most helpful in terms of describing what clinical supervision should be (Wright 1989).

Wright describes supervision as a process by which people together consider a piece of work in terms of 'what is happening and why, what was done and said, and how it was handled'. Wright goes on to describe the dynamic aspects of supervision in terms of thinking about the same piece of work to see if it could have been dealt with differently. Defined in these terms, supervision is seen as a collaborative venture in which the practitioner spends time, with at least one other person, reviewing what they are doing with a client and considering if what they are doing is in the best interests of the client. They also review how and if things might have been done differently. The process should be conducted without censure. In many respects the relationship between a supervisor and a supervisee should mirror the relationship between a client and a therapist. It must be collaborative. The significant players must have shared aims and agreed outcomes. There must be equality in the relationship.

Within nursing, this type of supervision is not a common feature of practice, although it does occur in some settings. Most commonly the kind of supervision described above is a feature of mental health services where multidisciplinary working has resulted in contact between nurses and social workers or psychotherapists – groups where clinical supervision is more firmly established. There are, however, areas in which clinical supervision is a well-established working practice. Kohner (1994), has collated information about how supervision is practised in a variety of health settings. These include acute and community services, demonstrating the possibility of establishing clinical supervision in these areas. On the basis of the information gathered in her review, Kohner identifies a number of practical guidelines that can be used to form a framework for the establishment of clinical supervision. This framework, although clearly aimed at encouraging organisational change, can be used by individuals who are seeking to ensure they access clinical supervision.

Kohner's first principle is that those participating in supervision have a shared understanding of its purpose, role and function. In the case of the practitioner of cognitive behaviour therapy, the function of the supervision will be to ensure that the practitioner is meeting the needs of the client in a way that is both ethical and efficient. The practitioner who becomes a supervisee, must be prepared to consider the effects of their practice and, if necessary, to change some aspects of it. As such, the function of supervision is to make sure that the therapy is being conducted in a way that has the client's needs as paramount. This will be discussed in more detail below.

Kohner also identifies the need for supervisors to be properly trained and have the ability to meet the needs of the supervisee. This is an important consideration for workers who intend to practise cognitive behaviour therapy. They must ensure that they are supervised by someone who him/herself has experience of using the therapy. It is not sufficient to seek supervision from an individual who is experienced only with working with the particular client group. They must have, in addition, experience and training in the use of cognitive behaviour therapy so that they can ensure that the practitioner is using the most effective tools to help the client change.

Hawkins and Shohet (1989) describe supervision as a way of helping the therapist to sustain a positive therapeutic relationship, particularly when there are issues in the relationship which mitigate against this. Supervision is described as doing this in a number of ways. For example:

- It helps in avoiding overinvolvement.
- It can provide an overview that ensures good practice and ethical issues are given due regard.
- It encourages creative thinking.
- It can take the heat out of situations, if the therapist feels that the client seems to disable the therapeutic process by their responses.

The therapeutic relationship is an interactive one in which both parties have an agenda. It is the responsibility of the therapist to recognise and be aware of their own agenda. In doing this, it should not impinge negatively on the therapeutic relationship. The purpose of supervision is to highlight the therapist's agenda and to offer him or her an opportunity to work on it actively, ensuring that it does not spill over into the therapeutic relationship thus hijacking the potential for the client's needs to be met. It should be an ongoing process because, as the therapist encounters new clients with different problems, so their own concerns, fears, difficulties and unresolved issues may come to the fore once again. Supervision can also help to highlight what motivates a person to be in a helping relationship with another person to whom they bear no relationship.

Hawkins and Shohet (1989) identify wanting to help as equivalent to needing to help. If the therapist needs to help, where does the need come from? How will they ensure that this need does not become the primary need in the therapeutic relationship? Heron (1990) describes the helper who is compulsive in their role, their need to help outweighing the needs of the clients to be helped. In such cases the therapeutic endeavour is based on the needs of the therapist, rather than those of the client. There are many examples of people who work in the so-called caring professions and appear to immerse themselves completely in their work. Yet when you look closely at their family and close relationships, it often becomes apparent that they are neglectful of these. For these people, it may be too painful to be responsive to the needs of their loved ones and so they compensate for the guilt they feel about this by becoming over-involved in the work they are doing with a particular client. Compulsive helpers work too hard. They see too many clients and are driven to keep going at all costs. For such therapists, the process of supervision will help to identify the source of their need and how they can meet their needs in another way.

Supervision is vital in dealing with the psychological baggage that a therapist brings to their work. It is also an important way to monitor the technical competence of the therapist. Heron identifies the unskilled therapist as one in need of supervision. When a therapy, such as cognitive behaviour therapy, is being used, there is the potential for the practitioner to dabble in techniques with which they are not competent or familiar. There is a huge array of techniques that the cognitive behavioural practitioner can use and this variety can be overwhelming. Through supervision, the practitioner can check out any concerns s/he may have about the use of any techniques s/he intends to use. It is for this reason that supervision should be conducted with a therapist who is skilled in the practice of cognitive behavioural techniques.

The process of supervision mirrors the therapeutic process. With both, there must be a willingness to participate. To prepare and to make use of what comes out of the process. In preparing for supervision, you, the therapist (supervisee), should spend time reflecting on the work you are engaged in with your clients. You should particularly note the thoughts and feelings you have about clients before the session starts. Do you get a sinking feeling before a particular client arrives, or what do you feel when someone cancels their appointment?

In preparation for supervision, you should consider if there are any techniques and tools you are using with which you are not familiar. You should be prepared to state clearly what your formulation is and how that is reflected by the work you are doing with the client. Have you obtained consent or are you assuming that because the person comes back to see you they are implying consent? Is implied consent sufficient? Supervision is a good opportunity to consider what the ethical dilemmas that arise from particular pieces of work may be.

When things do not go as planned

A crucial element of cognitive behaviour therapy is its transportability. It can be applied to work with a whole range of difficulties that a person may experience. These need not be mental health problems but include: physical health problems, for example, the treatment of chronic pain (Keefe et al. 1992); lifestyle problems, for example, social skills deficits (Williams 1986); relationship difficulties (Epstein et al. 1988); and anger management (Novaco 1975). The list of its applications is much longer than this and, by looking at the contents of any text about the practice of cognitive behaviour therapy, the range of situations to which it can be applied will be immediately apparent.

In many of these texts there will be evidence of the effectiveness of the approach in enabling people to overcome their difficulties. Part of this effectiveness should be attributed to the flexibility of the therapy. In assisting people to think about their difficulties, the cognitive behaviour therapist uses the technique of reframing. This has been described above as a process whereby the client is encouraged to think of an alternative interpretation of events, which s/he considers as negative. By doing this, the person is encouraged to minimise 'barriers' to change, and thereby maximise success and opportunities. Clearly this has to be done in a realistic way that conveys to the person that there will be occasions when things do not go quite as s/he had planned. The important lesson to pass on to the client is that unplanned things happen. S/he should not think of this as evidence that s/he is not progressing or that s/he cannot be helped by the therapy.

Unplanned events should be worked with and viewed as providing real opportunities for the client to practise his or her skills. They are excellent opportunities for the therapist to encourage generalisation of the various skills the client has learnt. If the unplanned event happens when the person is supported in a therapeutic relationship, then s/he has an opportunity to try out a different response to the situation.

It is this aspect of cognitive behaviour therapy that gives it face validity. Practitioners of the therapy must have a realistic view of people's lives. They need to recognise that people will face stressful events. They will have to cope with changes in their lives, they will have to cope with loss and bereavement. The timing of stressful life events cannot be planned – a difficulty may be encountered very soon after the person is discharged from therapy, or it may happen some time later. Whenever it does, the skills the person has acquired during his or her time in therapy will be invaluable to them. If the person is able to use these skills, s/he will be able to think of the events in a realistic way, a way which should help him or her to avoid a crisis.

Preparing for when things do not go as planned is variously labelled as relapse prevention, generalisation, and maintenance or inoculation training. The specific details of these aspects of the therapeutic episode are different but behind them lies the principle that, during therapy, a client should be given every opportunity to practise what s/he would do if things do not go as they planned.

How does nursing practice reflect elements of cognitive behaviour therapy?

Roper et al. (1980) designed a model of nursing to reflect British nursing practice in the early 1980s. Many of its elements reflect aspects of the process involved in the practice of cognitive behaviour therapy. There is some shared perspective between the two disciplines.

Earlier work by Orlando (1961) in the USA identified the process of nursing as a problem-solving activity which is deliberate, self-correcting and thoughtful. Over the last 20 years nursing has been increasingly defined as a process based on a human relationship, in which the development of the relationship is fundamental to the outcome. The importance of developing a trusting relationship will be emphasised throughout this book. The skills required to develop such a relationship are fundamental both to the practice of nursing and for those practising cognitive behaviour therapy. Relationships are defined throughout this text as a core element of cognitive behaviour therapy.

Roper conceptualised the role of the nurse as a helper (Roper 1976). Chapter 2 of this book outlines the various forms of help giving. It identifies helping as fundamental to cognitive behaviour therapy. The strategies identified in this book are all ways of helping the client to overcome their difficulties. Roper defined the task of nurses as that of a helper, with the aim of helping their clients to prevent, solve, alleviate or cope with actual or potential problems.

Nurses are considered to have a role to play in all aspects of health and ill health. In their role as health educators, they work with clients to prevent problems occurring. In their role as providers of health care, they work with clients to ensure the person maximises their potential to self-care (World Health Assembly 1989). Cognitive behaviour therapy has been shown to be effective not only in alleviating problems but also in preventing problems. In this respect the nurse who considers using cognitive behaviour therapy will already be familiar with the notion of assisting and enabling people both to deal with problems and to prevent problems from occurring. Nursing, as defined by Roper, is not about curing individuals, rather it is about enabling people to cope with their situation. This is a perspective that is familiar to those who practise cognitive behaviour therapy and is one of the reasons why preparing for unplanned events is identified as a major theme in this text.

The Roper–Logan–Tierney model defines nursing as a staged process that begins with assessment, an ongoing and active process through which problems are defined. These may be either actual or potential problems. Some will be amenable to intervention, some will not. The nurse must be able to discriminate between those problems that can be worked with and those which need to be referred on. This mirrors the times in therapy when recognising the limits of your own competence is crucial, if the client's best interests are to be served. Clearly, this skill is considered to be inherent in nursing practice and is identified as such in the United Kingdom Central Council for Nursing and Midwifery and Health Visiting (UKCC) (1992) Code of Conduct (Rule 18). This capacity, to discriminate what constitutes a real problem from a potential problem, what is amenable to therapy and what is better treated in another way, is an advanced skill, which develops through a process of reflection and accurate feedback during supervision. Without this feedback the needs of the therapist/nurse, rather than the client, can become pre-eminent.

Post Registration Education and Practice (PREP) aims to ensure that registered nurses develop their professional knowledge and competence. PREP identifies five categories of appropriate study for registered nurses; empowering consumers of health care is one of these. Empowerment is achieved in a setting where an individual or a group is encouraged to set their own goals. Goal setting is considered as a collaborative action for the nurse. It is also important for the cognitive behaviour therapist. Both practitioners, therefore, hold partnership and collaboration as defining features of the relationship they have with clients. The skills needed to ensure their presence in a therapeutic relationship are common features of both nurses and cognitive behaviour therapists.

Conclusions

Many of the words used in Rule 18 to describe the practice of nursing could equally be used to describe the practice of a cognitive behaviour therapist. It describes nursing as enabling and helpful. Practitioners of nursing require good communication skills. They must be able to identify needs and to assist people to move from a position of dependence to a point of independence. Nursing is described as a problem-solving activity that is conducted within a therapeutic relationship. Much of this could be a description of the process of cognitive behaviour therapy – the crucial omission being the philosophy that underpins the practice of this process. This text seeks to introduce the reader to this philosophy, it is written from the perspective that many of the skills necessary to practice cognitive behaviour therapy are already features of Registered Nurse practice.

References

Bandura, A. (1977) **Social Learning Theory**. Englewood Cliffs, NJ: Prentice Hall.

Beck, A.T. (1967) **Depression: Clinical, Experimental and Theoretical Perspectives**. New York: Hoeber.

Beck, A.T. (1976) **Cognitive Therapy and the Emotional Disorders**. New York: International University Press.

Beck, A.T. and Emery, G. (1985) **Anxiety Disorders and Phobias: A Cognitive Perspective**. New York: Basic Books.

Dryden, W. and Golden, W. (1986) **Cognitive Behavioural Approaches to Psychotherapy**. London: Harper and Row.

Dryden, W. and Rentoul, R. (1991) **Adult Clinical Problems: A Cognitive–Behavioural Approach**. London: Routledge.

Ellis, A. (1962) **Reason and Emotion in Psychotherapy**. New York: Lyle Stuart.

Epstein, N., Schlesinger, S. and Dryden, W. (1988) **Cognitive Behavioral Therapy with Families**. New York: Brunner/Mazel.

Faugier, J. and Butterworth, T. (1993) **Clinical Supervision: A Position Paper**. Manchester: The University of Manchester Press.

Gilbert, P. (1993) **Counselling for Depression**. London: Sage.

Hawkins, P. and Shohet, R. (1989) **Supervision in the Helping Professions**. Milton Keynes: Open University Press.

Heron, J. (1990) **Helping the Client. A Creative Practical Guide**. London: Sage.

Keefe, F., Dunsmore, J. and Burnett, R. (1992) Behavioural and cognitive–behavioural approaches to chronic pain: recent advances and future directions. **Journal of Consulting and Clinical Psychology** 60, 528–536.

Kelly, G. (1955) **The Psychology of Personal Construct Theory**. New York: Norton.

Kohner, N. (1994) **Clinical Supervision in Practice**. London: Kings Fund Centre.

Mahoney, M.J. (1993) Theoretical developments in cognitive psychotherapies. **Journal of Consulting and Clinical Psychology** 61, 187–193.

Marshall, S. (1992) A comparison of self instructional training and modelling for teaching an abstract task. **Mental Handicap** 20, 149–153.

Meichenbaum, D. (1977) **Cognitive Behavior Modification: An Integrative Approach**. New York: Pelum.

Novaco, R. (1975) **Anger Control: The Development and Evaluation of an Experimental Treatment**. Lexington: Heath and Company.

Orlando, I. (1961) **The Dynamic Nurse–Patient Relationship**. New York: Putman.

Robins, C.J. and Hayes, A.M. (1993) An appraisal of cognitive therapy. **Journal of Consulting and Clinical Psychology** 61, 203–214.

Rogers, C.R. (1967) **On Becoming a Person. A Therapist's View of Psychotherapy.** London: Constable.

Roper, N. (1976) **Clinical Experience in Nurse Education.** Edinburgh: Churchill Livingstone.

Roper, N., Logan, W. and Tierney, A. (1980) **The Elements of Nursing.** Edinburgh: Churchill Livingstone.

Rotter, J.B. and Hochreich, D.J. (1975) **Personality.** Glenorew: Scott Foreshaw.

Pavlov, I. (1927) **Conditioned Reflexes.** New York: Oxford University Press.

Tolman, E.C. (1932) **Purpose Behaviour in Animals and Men.** New York: Appleton.

United Kingdom Central Council for Nursing and Midwifery and Health Visiting (1990) **The Report of the Post Registration Education and Practice Project.** London: UKCC.

United Kingdom Central Council for Nursing and Midwifery and Health Visiting (1992) **Code of Professional Conduct.** London: UKCC.

Whitman, T., Spence, B. and Maxwell, S. (1987) A comparison of external and self instructional teaching formats with mentally retarded adults in vocational settings. **Applied Research in Developmental Disabilities** 8, 371.

Williams, J.H. (1986) Social skills and depression. In Hollin, C.R. and Trower, P. (eds) **Handbook of Social Skills Training.** Oxford: Pergamon.

World Health Assembly (1989) **Handbook of Resolutions and Decisions of the World Health Assembly and the Executive Board.** Geneva: WHO.

Wright, H. (1989) **Groupwork: Perspectives and Practice.** Oxford: Scutari Press.

Further reading

Persons, J. (1989) **Cognitive Therapy in Practice: A Case Formulation Approach.** New York: W.W. Norton.

Trower, P., Casey, A. and Dryden, W. (1988) **Cognitive Behavioural Counselling in Action.** London: Sage.

Dryden, W. and Rentoul, R. (1991) **Adult Clinical Problems: A Cognitive Behavioural Approach.** London: Routledge.

Feindler, E.L. and R.B. Ecton (1986) **Adolescent Anger Control: Cognitive Behavioural Techniques.** New York: Pergamon Press.

All of these texts give good illustrations of the range of uses to which cognitive behaviour therapy can be put. They all make reference to the seminal texts by Beck, Ellis and Meichenbaum, which are referenced in the preceding text.

SECTION 2

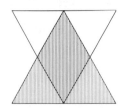

Applying Principles in Practice

SECTION 2

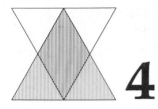

4

Naming the Problem
Assessment and formulation

Andy Farrington and Anni Telford

Key issues

- Therapeutic relationships
- Client/therapist alliance
- Models of assessment
- Behavioural and cognitive assessment
- Assessment style
- Suitability and incompatibility
- Supervision concepts and process

Introduction

In this chapter the reader will see the way in which initial therapeutic relationships are developed in cognitive behaviour therapy, particularly the processes involved and key techniques that enable the processes. Several models of assessment are then considered to illustrate cognitive behavioural assessment and problem formulation. Obviously not all assessments go well, therefore, issues surrounding the outcome of assessment, suitability for treatment and selection of the appropriate strategy will be discussed.

The chapter concludes by considering the function of clinical supervision as a method of maintaining objectivity and developing a problem-solving approach to difficult issues.

Relationships

Developing a good, sound therapeutic relationship that is built on trust and understanding is crucial to assessment and formulation in cognitive behaviour therapy. If the client is not engaged and committed to therapy from the outset, the future of the relationship is usually bleak and fraught with difficulties. Persuading the client at a later stage that therapy will be beneficial is especially problematic when an underpinning, quality relationship is absent.

Most approaches to therapy emphasise the importance of the client–therapist relationships as central in effecting cognitive and behavioural change (Schaap et al. 1993). Clearly the better the relationship, the more open the person being helped is about the thoughts and feelings that are occurring. The person is also more likely to explore these thoughts and feelings more deeply with the therapist, and to listen fully and act upon advice offered to him or her by the therapist.

Goldstein and Myers (1988) describe a therapeutic relationship as one in which feelings of liking are exhibited, respect and trust by the client toward the therapist are reciprocated by the therapist and suggests that several relationship-enhancing methods exist, which provide a framework for the improvement in the quality of the relationship, ensuring positive client change (see Figure 4.1).

The relationship-enhancing techniques can be divided into three areas of focus, those that deal with increasing the attraction of the client toward the therapist, those that deal with the characteristics of the therapist and those that consider expectancies and non-verbal communications.

Attractiveness

Client modelling

Modelling or observational learning can be used to expose the client to a person, i.e. a model or stooge, who role-plays the part of a client who not only likes the therapist but says so in clear terms. This approach is sometimes called imitation and relies on statements about the therapist presented to the client, which focus on positive aspects of behaviour and cognitions.

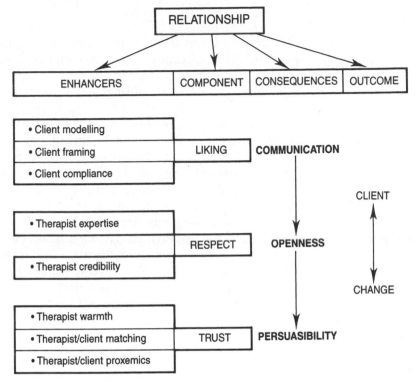

Figure 4.1 A framework for improving the quality of a therapeutic relationship [adapted from Goldstein and Myers (1988)].

An example of this is when a model makes a statement about the therapist like 'I'm finding it much easier to talk to you about my problems now that I have got over my initial anxiety about meeting you'.

Client framing

Framing the relationship consists simply of telling the client that they will like their therapist, describing to the client the positive characteristics of the therapist and providing clarification about what the client might reasonably anticipate will occur in the meetings with the therapist. Empirical work by Ford (1978), which examined the relationship between the client's perception of the therapeutic relationship and the behaviour therapist's behaviour, showed that a non-verbal style characterised by certainty, warmth, sincerity, relaxation, control and emotional responsiveness corresponded with positive client ratings, which were also a good predictor of treatment outcome.

Client compliance

To facilitate the client's commitment to therapy, it is useful to involve accomplices to persuade the client to conform to a majority decision or judgement, so, for example, using the peer pressure of a group to encourage a client to complete set tasks during initial assessment interviews.

Clearly the enhancing of a therapeutic relationship at the assessment stage is likely to prevent clients dropping out of treatment later on. However, factors that have been shown to be linked to clients' non-compliance with advice and directives include situations in which the therapist is too domineering and controlling, rejecting of the clients' opinions and in complete disagreement with the views of the client (Schaap et al. 1993). There is also a danger in the use of the term non-compliance in that it can suggest the negative image of a difficult client who is reactive, and resistant to assessment and therapy, and whilst change can be difficult for clients to undertake, several studies have shown that reactance in certain phases of treatment is in fact associated with a positive outcome (Orlinsky and Howard, 1978; Schaap and Schippers, 1986; Tennen et al. 1981).

Characteristics of the therapist

Therapist expertise

Expertise as well as status can be conveyed by several methods; the actual physical surroundings that the therapist works within can convey a clear message about the position of the therapist within an organisation. For example, a dingy poorly lit office with broken furniture and in need of a good coat of paint can usually be interpreted as the therapist having a low priority in terms of being 'looked after' by the organisation.

Trappings such as the title used by the therapist, nationally and internationally recognised qualifications, type and number of books on the bookshelf, behaviour of the therapist and the way in which s/he dresses, all add up to the big picture of the status and expertise of the therapist as perceived by the client. Expertise can also be conveyed by the therapist predicting symptoms that the client is likely to experience, for example, if a client describes having panic attacks, the therapist could suggest that the client may experience breathlessness, choking, palpitations and a dry throat.

Clinical competence can also be demonstrated by the therapist displaying self-assurance and taking the lead in situations when the client is hesitant. Research by Frank (1982) suggests that displaying appropriate books and certificates in fact does add to the overall picture of expertise, as well as the importance of the therapist's reputation, as a way of presenting self-confidence, which creates hope and positive expectations for the client. The client can then be assured that the therapist will do their utmost to help them overcome their difficulty.

Therapist credibility

Clearly, it is important that the therapist maintains an image of credibility in his or her working clinical practice. Credibility, which is an ability perceived by the client for the therapist to be knowledgeable about current and valid information, and to be motivated to communicate unbiased information, consists of:

- The expertise of the therapist as demonstrated by title, institutional affiliation and other aspects of academic and professional achievement.
- The reliability of the therapist as a source of information, which includes qualities such as being able to be depended upon, behaving in a predictable way and remaining consistent throughout the relationship.
- The motivations and intentions of the therapist, in other words, the interests of the client remain at the forefront of the relationship with the client, and are not put into a position of secondary or less importance.
- The dynamism of the therapist, demonstrated by the appearance of self-confidence, assertive abilities, attention to detail and the proactive manner in which s/he deals with issues and the client.

Several non-verbal cues have also been associated with success in creating the right image as a therapist; for example, rapid and fluent speech, a standard accent, speech that is not too loud or too soft, and good eye contact (Cappella and Street 1985; Street and Hopper 1982; Patterson 1982).

Therapist warmth

This aspect of the relationship is concerned with communicating warmth unconditionally and without restriction, including the notion that there should be a deep respect for the client's worth as a person and his or her rights as a free individual. The client needs to be free of constraint to be him/herself, even if that means regressing, being defensive or even disliking or helping the therapist. Warmth and humour have, however, been argued only to be effective if the therapist is able to structure sessions and have clear directives (Alexander et al. 1976).

In addition to warmth, the issue of empathy is also important in the construction of the therapeutic alliance. Truax and Carkhuff (1967) describe a five-point empathy scale from very low (level 1) to very high (level 5). The range of levels moves from the low, in which the therapist takes no notice of the communicative and behavioural expressions of the client, to the high, when the therapist responds accurately to the client's superficial and deep feelings. The therapist at this point is often described as being in tune with or on the same wavelength as the client.

Empathy, whilst in itself is not sufficient for positive therapeutic change, is recognised within many psychotherapeutic schools as being one of the key elements in the creation of the therapeutic alliance and a strategy which is likely to produce increased client self-disclosure (Hopkinson et al. 1981).

One final aspect of this part of the characteristics of the therapist is self-disclosure. In the course of therapy, it is common for the client to reveal information about him/herself, which concerns his or her personal needs, problems, history and relationships, particularly as s/he becomes more comfortable and at ease with the therapist.

The task of the therapist is to respond by offering facilitative conditions and reciprocating self-disclosure by disclosing such information as views about the client, reactions to the unfolding situation or information of a personal nature. Obviously the idea of the therapist talking about their own personal issues to the client needs careful handling, especially timing of the delivery and the type of information that is appropriate to reveal. It can be assumed that, if as suggested previously, client self-disclosure is an important aspect of therapy, then therapist self-disclosure in line with the reciprocity principle will lead to increased client self-disclosure. However, Curtis (1982) showed that therapist self-disclosure resulted in lower client empathy and trust, and lower perceptions of therapist competence.

Expectancies and non-verbal communications

Therapist–client matching

Whilst matching the therapist/client is not a prerequisite for the therapeutic relationship, several features exist that have been shown to be contributing factors in ensuring that good fit occurs. Setting ground rules from the outset and establishing the do's and don'ts is particularly important, as is anticipation of client change and positive results from meetings.

In addition, similar social, cultural, racial and economic backgrounds, language use and social awareness have all been shown to support a positive therapeutic relationship.

Therapist–client proxemics

Spatial awareness is often neglected in discussions about the developing of a good therapeutic relationship. Distance apart from the client as well as posture are important in fostering effective verbal com and particular attention needs to be paid to variables such cultural background, in which proximity needs to be adjuste ingly. Not every client is comfortable sitting 25–30 inches away from therapist, with the therapist leaning 20% towards the client and maintaining eye contact 90% of the time. In fact, there are many occasions in cognitive behavioural psychotherapy when emotions are elicited from the client and the therapist needs to move closer to the client who is upset or back from the client who is angry.

It has been argued recently that there is an increased activity by researchers and psychotherapists into the nature of common and non-specific factors in the therapeutic relationship. Common factors are considered to be those variables that are common across the board of a wide range of therapeutic interventions and styles. Non-specific factors are those that the therapist does not consider important within the context of the specific treatment strategy being used (Schaap et al. 1993).

Therapists using a cognitive behavioural approach, however, have until recently tended to dismiss or fail to consider the therapeutic relationship as having a bearing on therapy, and have assigned any reference to the therapeutic relationship as being non-specific (Schaap et al. 1993). The historical development of cognitive behavioural psychotherapy has been typified by a scant regard for the therapeutic relationship, with research focusing on the so-called active ingredient of the therapeutic process, the technique, rather than the construction of a client–therapist relationship.

Whilst the therapeutic relationship is now more likely to be in the spotlight of psychotherapy research generally, there continues to be minimal empirical research that examines the development of the therapeutic alliance in cognitive behaviour therapy. Morris and Suckerman (1974), for example, showed that, if a therapist engaged in therapy was perceived to be warm and friendly, then better outcome results from the client were seen when compared to a therapist who was cold. Clearly research of this nature is always going to be inelegant and questionable when reducing a complex phenomena to a two-dimensional position.

The use of contingency contracting in behavioural marital therapy, whereby the couple negotiate a contract in which specific change to behaviour and cognitions as desired by the other partner is drawn up, is common. Recent research by Schindler et al. (1983) suggests that couples who received contingency contracting and who showed success over a long term rated their therapists as being more empathic, directive and active. Similarly Bennun and Schindler (1988) in addition to Emmelkamp and Van der Hout (1983) found a significant correlation in their research between clinical outcome measures and therapeutic relationship in the treatment of patients with agoraphobia-type problems.

As suggested previously, if a client is not engaged and committed to therapy from the outset, the future of the relationship is bleak, but, in addition, it is also important to seek and gain informed consent from the client at the outset of therapy. This means:

- Providing a clear explanation to the client about the nature and outcome of assessment and evaluation.
- Describing the specific aims of treatment, the treatment option of choice and alternative treatment methods available.
- Communicating to the client the proven effectiveness of the treatment or the experimental nature of treatment, if new techniques are being used.

Consent may then be sought from the client to continue with therapy either explicitly in written form or by verbal agreement to attend for treatment.

In summary, traditional behaviour therapy has generally neglected the notion of the therapeutic alliance, especially the creation of a positive therapeutic relationship, and has concentrated its attention on the technique aspects of therapy delivery. Whilst several recent studies suggest the importance of research into the therapeutic relationship in cognitive behaviour therapy, it remains largely in the domain of a non-specific factor at present.

What is, however, becoming clear is that across psychotherapies, regardless of delivery style and underpinning philosophy, there is much to be gained from further research that considers the idea of common factors in therapy, particularly empirical analysis, which can best inform clinical practice.

The next section of this chapter will examine in detail the assessment and formulation process in cognitive behaviour therapy and present several models of assessment that have been tried and tested over many years.

Strategies

The initial assessment and formulation process in cognitive behaviour therapy is the foundation on which any treatment programme is built. Assessment is about gaining data from which conclusions can be drawn and the identification of variables impinging on the problem. Formulation is concerned with the decisions made about the nature of the client's problem, construction of a meaningful problem statement and selection of an intervention.

Faulty assessment and inaccurate problem identification is one of the main causes of treatment failure and there are two main questions that should be uppermost in the interviewer's mind at this point. The first is 'What is it that the client does and says to themselves that interferes with their lives?' Clearly assessment is concerned with both behaviours that the client is doing, such as avoiding going out alone or socialising, and also the internal cognitive dialogue that is occurring, such as 'if anyone sees me in this state they will think I'm mad'. The second is 'What are they failing to do and say, which, if present, would help them achieve their life goals?' For example, if a client with a social anxiety problem joined a social group, it would enable the client to meet others, or if a client said to him/herself that 'I've done this before successfully and can do it again with practice'.

The length of assessment and the time taken to obtain answers to the questions depends on the individual client's problems: a simple mono-symptomatic phobia may only take a matter of hours to assess, whereas a complex obsessive compulsive disorder can take anything from 2 to 10 hours to thoroughly assess. Whilst there are no hard and fast rules about assessment, the minimum period in which to gather sufficient quality information to formulate a clear picture of the problem should be in the region of at least 1–2 hours.

Complex problems do require many hours of assessment, perhaps two or more assessment appointments being required. It is, therefore, wise to plan ahead and book sufficient time in diaries, and accommodation for the period of the interview.

It is unethical, however, to collect excess information. Asking questions for the sake of it or to fill in time is costly in terms of the client's time, your time and NHS monies. Although all aspects of the client in his/her environment may and generally do require examination, even if only briefly to ascertain that it is not a problem area.

Forms and questionnaires used to excess are a poor substitute for a well-executed assessment interview, which can provide an ideal vehicle for establishing a good therapeutic relationship between the client and therapist on the way to the creation of a positive therapeutic alliance. Empathy, understanding and professional concern as described previously are also important issues during the first contact with the client, and may well determine a good outcome of treatment.

Before describing the elements which make up several models of behavioural and cognitive behavioural assessment, three case studies will be identified to illustrate the models.

Case illustrations

- Jennifer Bowles is a 62-year-old woman with an obsessive compulsive problem of multiple checking rituals.
- Paul Scott is a 25-year-old man who experiences anxiety and panic.
- Howard Jones is a 48-year-old man with depression and difficulty in mixing with people.

Models of assessment

Over the last 25 years, several models of behavioural and cognitive assessment have been developed, the most widely used with small variations being, for behavioural assessment, Kanfer and Saslow's (1969) seven-part analysis/plan (Model 1), and for behavioural and cognitive assessment, Lazarus's (1973) multimodal behavioural assessment (Model 2) and Lang's (1970) three-systems analysis (Model 3).

Behavioural assessment

Seven-part analysis

The first model originates from the work of Kanfer and Saslow (1969) and, as its name suggests, considers assessment in a seven-part plan, and focuses on the behavioural components of cognitive behavioural assessment.

1. Initial analysis of the problem situation

Particularly, is the behaviour an excess, a deficit or an asset? Frequency, intensity, duration and stimulus conditions are also considered at this point.

a. *Behavioural excess.* A class of related behaviours occurs and is described as problematic by the client or an informant because of excess in: (1) frequency; (2) intensity; (3) duration or (4) occurrence under conditions when its socially sanctioned frequency approaches zero. Compulsive handwashing, combativeness, prolonged excitement and sexual exhibitionism are examples of behavioural excess along one or another of these four dimensions. Less obvious, because they often do not constitute the major presenting complaint and appear only in the course of the behavioural analysis, are examples of socially unacceptable, solitary, affectionate or other private behaviours.

Mrs Bowles described multiple checking rituals lasting 8–9 hours per day of household items like food, the kettle, knives, scissors and cleaning agents to reassure herself that no harm could come to another person as a result of her negligence. She also chanted words aloud like 'salt, salt' up to 50 times before adding it to a meal in case she poisoned someone. From this example, it is clear that both duration and intensity values of the behaviour may jointly determine the characterisation of the behaviour as excessive.

b. *Behavioural deficit.* A class of responses is described as problematic by someone because it fails to occur: (1) with sufficient frequency; (2) with adequate intensity; (3) in appropriate form or (4) under socially expected conditions. Examples are: reduced social responsiveness (withdrawal); amnesias; fatigue syndromes; and restrictions in sexual or somatic function, e.g. impotence, writer's cramp. Other examples of behaviour deficits can be found in depressed clients who have no appropriate behaviour in a new social environment, e.g. after changes from a rural to an urban area, from marital to single status, or from one socioeconomic level to another. Clients typically described as inadequate are often found to have large gaps in their social or intellectual repertoire, which prevent appropriate actions.

Mrs Bowles complained of having little or no time to look after the house or her personal appearance because she was spending so much time checking.

c. *Behavioural assets.* Behavioural assets are non-problematic behaviours. What does the client do well? What are his/her adequate social behaviours? What are his/her special talents or assets? The content of life experiences that can be used to execute a therapeutic programme is unlimited. Any segment of the client's activities can be used as an arena for building up new behaviours. In fact, his/her natural work and play activities provide a better starting point for behaviour change than can ever be provided in a synthetic activity or relationship. For example, a person with musical talent, skill in a craft, physical skill or social appeal can be helped to use his/her strengths as vehicles for changing behaviour relationships, and for acquiring new behaviours in areas in which some successful outcomes are highly probable. While a therapeutic goal may ultimately be the acquisition of specific social or self-evaluative behaviour, the learning can be programmed with many different tasks and in areas in which the client has already acquired competence.

Mrs Bowles has successfully managed to hold down a part-time job as a nurse as well as being an active member of a local amateur dramatics group.

2. Clarification of the problem situation

a. Assign the classes of problematic responses to Group A behavioural excess or Group B behavioural deficit described above, as the assessment proceeds and clarity is achieved.
b. Which persons or groups object to these behaviours? Which persons or groups support them? Who persuaded or coerced the client to come to the clinician?

In the example of Mrs Bowles, her husband was starting to become alarmed and concerned at the amount of time his wife was taking to prepare meals, and the number of precautions and checks she was having to make. He attended the first assessment interview with his wife.

c. What consequences does the problem have for the client and for significant others? What consequences would removal of the problem have for the client or others?

   If Mrs Bowles did not have the problem with checking, it would free up to 8–9 hours in a day and enable her to increase her part-time hours at work and make a bigger financial contribution to the household.

d. Under what conditions do the problematic behaviours occur (biological, symbolic, social, vocational, etc.)?

   For Mrs Bowles the problem increases in severity if anyone visits the house or if she is tired from her part-time job.

e. What satisfaction would continue for the client if his/her problematic behaviour were sustained? What satisfactions would the client gain if, as a result of psychological intervention, his/her problematic behaviour were changed? What positive or aversive effects would occur for significant others if the client's problematic behaviour were changed? How would the client continue to live if therapy were unsuccessful, i.e. if no behaviour changed?

   Keeping the checking rituals going initially acts as a reassurance for Mrs Bowles, although this tends to diminish after about 2 hours.

f. What new problems in living would successful therapy pose for the client? What reinforcers are there?

g. To what extent is the client as a sole informant capable of helping in the development of a therapy programme?

   The questions raised here are derived from the assumption that maladjusted behaviour requires continued support. It cannot be banished from the client's life for all future circumstances. Change in it is related closely to the environment in which the person needs to live. Elimination of the problematic behaviour is also impossible as long as powerful, and often undefined, reinforcing events operate. The answers to the above questions can help to bring about an early decision about the optimal goals within practical reach of the clinician and within the inevitably fixed boundaries of the client's life pattern.

3. Motivational analysis

This part of the assessment is concerned with the question of what the potent reinforcers are.

a. How does the client rank various incentives in their importance to him/her? Basing judgement on the client's probable expenditure of time, energy or physical discomfort, which of the following reinforcing events are relatively most effective in initiating or maintaining his/her behaviour: achievement of recognition, sympathy, friendship, money, good health, sexual satisfaction, intellectual competence, social approval, work satisfaction, control over others, securing dependency, etc.?

b. How frequent and regular have been his/her successes with these reinforcers? What are his/her present expectations of success for each? Under what circumstances was reinforcement achieved for each of these incentives?

c. Under what specific conditions do each of these reinforcers arouse goal-directed behaviour (biological, symbolic, social, vocational)?

d. Do his/her actions in relation to those goals correspond with verbal statements? How does any definable discrepancy affect goals and procedures in therapy?

e. Which persons or groups have the most effective and widespread control over his/her current behaviour?

f. Can the client relate reinforcement contingencies to his/her own behaviour, or does s/he assign reinforcement to random uncontrollable factors, for example, superstitious behaviour, belief in luck, fate, miracles, etc.?

g. What are the major aversive stimuli for this client: (1) in immediate day-to-day life; and (2) in the future? Are there bodily sensations, conviction of illness or fears of illness that serve as important stimuli for change? What are his/her fears, the consequences that s/he avoids and dreads, the risks which s/he does not take?

h. Would a treatment programme require that the client give up current satisfactions associated with his/her problem, e.g. invalid status in the family or on the job; gratifications, possibly due to unemployment; life restrictions and special privileges justified by his/her 'nervous' status; illness as justification for failure to fulfil expectations of him/herself or others?

i. Which events of known reinforcing value can be utilised for learning new interpersonal skills or self-attitudes during treatment? In what areas and by what means can positive consequences be arranged to follow desired behaviours, replacing earlier aversive consequences.

4. Development analysis

What are the biological, sociological and behavioural changes?

a. Biological changes:

1. What are the limitations in the client's biological equipment that may affect current behaviour, e.g. defective vision and hearing; residuals of illnesses such as stroke, poliomyelitis, mononucleosis, glandular imbalances? How do these limitations initiate or maintain undesirable

behaviours, e.g. behavioural constrictions owing to fatigue, fear of overexertion, avoidance of social exposure of these deficits? Can the client's self-limiting expectations of the interfering consequences be changed?

Mrs Bowles has had a hysterectomy and suffered lacerated skull with some olfactory nerve damage.

2. When and how did biological deviations or limitations develop? What consequences did they have on his/her life pattern and on his/her self-attitudes? What was done about them, by whom? Has s/he developed specific consistent response patterns towards some body structure or function?
3. How do these biological conditions limit response to treatment or resolution of his/her problems?

b. *Sociological changes:*
1. What are the most characteristic features of the client's present sociological milieu (with regard to urban versus rural environment, religious affiliation, socioeconomic status, ethnic affiliation, educational–intellectual affiliation, etc.)? Are their attitudes congruent with this milieu? For instance, how is a college orientation of an adolescent accepted by his peer group in a different neighbourhood? How does the home and neighbourhood environment respond to a client's religious, social and sexual activities and fantasies?

Mrs Bowles lives in a three-bedroomed bungalow with her husband and has good links with the neighbours.

2. Have there been changes in this milieu which are pertinent to his/her current behaviour? If so, how long ago, how permanently, and under what conditions did such changes occur? What immediate consequences did they have for the behaviour of the client? For example, what impact on a wife did a husband's rapid promotion have? Or a marriage into different socioeconomic or religious group? Or a move from a rural southern community to an urban northern part of the United Kingdom?
3. Does the client view these changes as brought about by himself/herself, by significant persons or by fortuitous circumstances? What attitudes does s/he have about these changes?
4. Are the client's roles in various social settings congruent with one another? For example, is there role conflict between value systems of the client's early and adult social environments? Are there behavioural deficits owing to the changes, e.g. an inability to cope with new social demands, sexual standards or affectional requirements, associated with rapid acquisition or loss of wealth or geographic location? If the roles are incongruent, is incongruence among these roles pertinent to

his/her problem? Does the problematic behaviour occur in all or only some of these different settings?

5. How can identified sociological factors in the problematic behaviour be brought into relation with a treatment programme?

c. Behavioural changes:

1. Prior to the time of referral, did the client's behaviour show deviations in behaviour patterns compared with developmental and social norms? If so, what was the nature of changes in social behaviours, in routine self-care behaviours, in verbal statements towards self and others? Under what conditions were these changes first noted?

2. Do identified biological, social or sociological events in the client's life seem relevant to these behavioural changes?

3. Were these changes characterised by: (a) emergence of new behaviours; (b) change in intensity or frequency of established behaviours; (c) non-occurrence of previous behaviours?

4. Under what conditions and in which social settings were these behavioural changes first noted? Have they extended to other social settings since the problematic behaviour was first noted?

5. Were the behavioural changes associated with the client's exposure to significant individuals or groups from whom s/he learned new patterns of reinforcement and the behaviour necessary to achieve them? Can the problematic behaviours be traced to a model in the client's social environment from whom s/he has learned these responses?

5. Analysis of self-control

How can the client's self-controlling behaviour be used in the treatment programme?

a. In what situations can the client control those behaviours that are problematic? How does s/he achieve such control, by manipulation of self or others?

   Mrs Bowles is able to control the problem at work by saying to herself that she will lose her job if she checks at work.

b. Have any of the problematic behaviours been followed by aversive consequences, e.g. social retribution, jail, ostracism, probation, etc.? Have these consequences reduced the frequency of the problematic behaviour or only the conditions under which it occurs? Have these events modified the client's self-controlling behaviour?

c. Has the client acquired some measure of self-control in avoiding situations that are conducive to the execution of his/her problematic behaviour? Does s/he do this by avoidance or by substitution of alternative instrumental behaviours leading to similar satisfactions?

d. Is there correspondence between the client's verbalised degree of self-control and observations by others? Can the client match his/her behaviour to his/her intentions?

e. What conditions, persons or reinforcers tend to change his/her self-controlling behaviour, e.g. a child behaves acceptably at school but not at home, or vice versa?

f. To what extent can the client's self-controlling behaviour be used in a treatment programme? Is constant supervision of drug administration necessary to supplement self-control, for example?

6. Analysis of relevant social relationships

a. Who are the most significant people in the client's current environment? To which persons or groups is s/he most responsive? Who facilitates constructive behaviours? Who provokes antagonistic or problematic behaviours? Can these relationships be categorised according to dimensions that clarify the client's behavioural patterns, e.g. does a client respond in a submissive or hostile way to all older men/younger women?

b. In these relationships, by use of what reinforcers do the participants influence each other? For example, analysis may reveal a father who always bails out a delinquent son whose public punishment would be embarrassing to the father. Is the cessation of positive reinforcement or onset of punishment clearly signalled?

c. What does the client expect of these people in words and in action? On what does s/he base his/her verbal expectations?

d. What do these people expect of the client? Is there consistency between the client's and others' expectations for him/her?

e. How can the people who can influence the client participate in treatment?

7. Assessment of the sociocultural and physical environment

a. What are the norms in the client's social milieu for the behaviours about which there is a complaint?

b. Are these norms similar in the various environments in which the client interacts, e.g. home and school, friends and parents, work and social milieu, etc.? If not, what are the major differences in behaviours supported in one but not the other environments?

c. In which portion of the environment is the client's problematic behaviour most apparent, most troublesome or most accepted? Can the congruence of several environments be increased or can the client be helped by removal from dissonant environments? Does his/her milieu permit or discourage self-evaluation?

d. Does his/her milieu regard psychological procedures as appropriate for helping him/her solve his/her problem? Is there support in his/her milieu for the changes in attitudes and values that successful psychotherapy may require?

In the case summary of the assessment of Jennifer Bowles, she is a 62-year-old woman with an obsessive compulsive checking problem of 32 years duration due to the fear and anxiety of causing injury or harm to others by neglect. Onset of the problem followed what she described as 'a mental breakdown' at secondary school. She now spends 8–9 hours every day checking (mainly in the home) food, kitchen items, disinfectants and cleaning agents, light switches, taps, doors, waste bins, knobs and buttons in the kitchen and gas pipes. Outside the home she checks gates, people crossing the road and shelves in shops. She talked off the point at times during the first assessment interview and checked items such as the door of the office being shut, and that she had been given information which she understood and was 'correct' by repeating back aloud the words of the therapist as a checking behaviour.

Behavioural and cognitive assessment _____

Multimodal behavioural assessment

The second model of assessment comes from the work of Lazarus (1973), which bears much similarity to that of Kanfer and Saslow (1969) and is easily remembered by the mnemonic BASIC-ID (B – Behaviour; A – Affect; S – Sensations; I – Imagery; C – Cognition; I – Interpersonal relationships; D – Drugs).

The second illustrative case in summary using this assessment model is as follows.

Behaviour

Paul Scott is a 25-year-old man with a 2-year history of feelings of anxiety and panic, due to the fear of dying from a heart attack or stroke, which results in the avoidance of being alone in situations such as when shopping, and travelling on buses and tube trains. He also avoids any form of exertion or physical exercise.

Affect

At interview, he appeared worried about his problem and how it was starting to have an impact on his students' studies. There was no evidence of clinical depression, although he was tearful on occasions.

Sensations

He described listening to his heart beating to make sure it was all right, and feeling for and checking his pulse every 15–20 minutes when he is anxious. He experiences palpitations, dry throat and a feeling that his legs are going to 'suddenly give way' as he says.

Imagery

He sometimes experiences a future prediction image in which he sees himself dying alone of a heart attack in an open park with no one about to help him. This occurs 2–3 times a month.

Cognition

His internal dialogue consists of negative self-talk, particularly when he has exerted himself such as 'I must check my pulse to make sure I'm not having a heart attack ... my pulse seems far too quick ... I must be having a heart attack ... there is no one here to help me ... I must get myself to the nearest hospital for a check up ... my father had a heart attack when he was my age'.

Interpersonal relationships

He lives in a one-bedroomed flat with his wife, has no links with the neighbours and only socialises with two close friends that he has known since primary school.

Drugs

He is using a minor tranquilliser prescribed by his general practitioner for panic attacks.

The final model of assessment is probably the most commonly used in cognitive behavioural assessment, and combines the elements of behaviour, physiology and cognition to create a model that considers all aspects of the client rather than component parts.

Three-systems analysis

The third model of assessment originated from the work of Lang (1970) and is based on the idea that fear is best construed as a set of three loosely coupled components: behaviour, physiology and cognition.

As is clear, both Lazarus (1973) and Lang (1970) provide a model of assessment that includes elements of Kanfer and Saslow's (1969) seven-part plan, with the addition of a cognitive component to make up what has now come to be described as a cognitive behavioural assessment.

Whilst the behavioural and physiological parts of the assessment have been described elsewhere, the purpose of this part of the assessment is to establish the client's thoughts and perceptions before, during and after any event or set of stimuli, and, by so doing, identify the misconceptions and thinking style of the client, which is preventing them from achieving their life goals.

The case of Howard Jones who has a problem of mixing with people and depression, will serve to illustrate this part of the cognitive behavioural assessment interview.

The main faulty thinking styles to look for include:

1. Dichotomous reasoning (thinking in black and white terms)
    e.g. 'I knew the minute that woman didn't speak to me it was going to be a bad day.'
2. Personalisation (blaming yourself for something which is not your fault)
    e.g. 'It's my fault my wife left me.'
3. Mind reading (believing you know what others think of you)
    e.g. 'They were all looking at me and must have thought I was crazy.'
    'They all thought I was stupid.'
4. Arbitrary inference (making a decision on something where there is either none or contrary evidence)
    e.g. 'She didn't call therefore I must have upset her.'
    'My boss only said I'd done a good job to please me.'
5. Overgeneralisation (taking one piece of evidence as an indicator towards other unrelated situations or circumstances)
    e.g. 'I failed that exam – I'm an idiot.'
    'They all hate me.'
6. Magnification (or awfulisation) (making things out to be much worse than they really are)
    e.g. 'It was really terrible, I thought I was dying.'
    'I can't stand it when I get anxious, it's awful.'
7. Minimisation (turning success/achievement/personal assets into nothing)
    e.g. 'Oh, it was nothing really, anyone could have done it.'
    'You think my shirt's nice? It's terrible really.'
8. Labelling (attaching general labels to oneself)
    e.g. 'I'm useless.'
    'I can't cope.'
    'I'm just a depressive.'
    'I'm a hopeless case.'

The therapist attempts to perceive the style and frequency of the client's dialogue and its relationship to their behaviour.

There are a variety of questions and techniques one can use in attempting to elicit cognitions from a client. Questions might include:

- 'What were you thinking about just before this?'
- 'What were you thinking about during it?'
- 'What were you thinking about immediately after that happened?'
- 'What was going on in your head/were you telling yourself?'
- 'What do you think they thought about you?'
- 'What does that mean about you as a person/daughter/wife/husband, etc.?'
- 'Why is that important to you?'
- 'What images/pictures did you have at the time?'
- 'What did you think was going to happen to you at that point/next?'
- 'Why did that frighten/anger/depress you?'
- 'What was it about the situation that frightened/angered/depressed you?'
- 'What does that imply?'

Some clients find it extremely difficult to give a clear picture of their thoughts and a variety of techniques can be used to help them:

1. Imaginal technique. Ask the client to close their eyes, and think back and imagine the last time they were in the situation. Then use questions as required.
2. Behavioural test/task. Ask the client to perform the actions that usually occur when the thoughts are present. For example, ask a person with agoraphobia to go to the shops and then either go with them and use questions from above as required, or ask them to 'talk' their thoughts into a dictaphone as they go along.
3. Incident analysis. Ask the client to talk you through a typical situation in great detail. Use questions as required, including: 'What were you thinking then/at that point?'.
4. Video tape. If a client still cannot produce cognitions after a behavioural test, film them performing the same, then watch it with them, asking: 'What do you think you were thinking at that point?'. Stop the film and let them answer.
5. Essay. This is useful for clients with low self-confidence/self-worth/depression. Ask them to write an essay (one side of A4) about themselves.
6. Labels. These again are useful for clients with low self-worth/depression. Have 50 cards with adjectives on saying 'wonderful', 'useless', 'stupid', 'clever', i.e. 25 positive and 25 negative. Ask them to pick out those that apply to them.
7. Client in the pocket technique. If all else fails try this technique: 'My last client was very much like you and had a similar problem, s/he used to think [such and such] in similar situations, does that sound like you?'

Use your clinical experience to feed to the client some examples of what clients with similar problems might be thinking. Beware of leading the client too much. If they say 'No, that doesn't sound like me', accept it and try some other approach.

Assessment style

When interviewing, it is useful to become familiar with a style that is comfortable to use and easy to remember. One such style is that of scan, select and focus:

- Scan – involves looking broadly at all times of information received.
- Select – identifies the pieces of information that are appropriate and relevant.
- Focus – examine, by close questioning, the relevant and appropriate areas.

When jargon words or general terms are used, ask exactly what is meant by them. Similarly, try to make sure that the language, phrases and expressions used are familiar to the client. Use reflective feedback to make sure you have got your facts right, i.e. simply rephrase the information and return it to the client to ensure s/he agrees. Occasionally pause and summarise what information you have so far to ensure accuracy. Be warm and open, and use self-disclosure where appropriate, i.e. 'Yes, I've had something similar to that happen to me'.

Avoid putting words into the client's mouth by using leading questions. Instead, use open questions, e.g. leading question: 'Do you feel depressed?'; open question: 'How is your mood?' If you fail to elicit factual responses by using open questions, use more closed ones – but go back to open questions as soon as possible.

Clients often feel they are the only people who have ever experienced problems. Let them know they are not alone by referring to other people, i.e. 'Yes, we've seen many people who feel like that/have experienced that'.

If a strong emotion is expressed, i.e. anger, panic, agitation, distress, tears, etc., respond appropriately with care, warmth, patience and gentle questioning. Reduce excess emotion then examine how it arose and its relevance. If emotion prevents a certain line of questioning, then approach from another angle or slow down the information-gathering process.

Periodically reflect on your own performance and examine it as objectively as possible. What could be improved? What could be omitted? How are your social skills?

See relatives, friends and appropriate others to verify and enlarge on the client's description. Relatives can also be affected by the client's problem; however, they can also make excellent helpers. Remember that you need the client's consent to talk to any others and also the consent of the client to disclose any information to a partner/relative/friend.

At the end of the assessment, you should be able to:

- Write an assessment report.
- Describe, with measurement, the client's problem.
- Describe, in detail, the objectives.
- Offer a plan of management.
- Set an appropriate evaluation date.

In the case of Howard Jones the following illustrates the kind of information that is needed for an assessment report.

Mr Jones identified his main problem as a 2-year history of difficulty in initiating and maintaining a conversation with females and males of all ages, but especially people who were strangers and women. This was due to anxiety and feelings of panic, which resulted in the avoidance of mixing with people and interacting socially. As a direct result of the problem, he panics on average twice per week, which he describes as shaking hands, stomach turning over and headaches. He daily avoids talking to people at work and socially. The usual pattern when he attempts to initiate a conversation is that he 'dries up, becomes embarrassed, thinks to himself "I'm behaving like an idiot", and escapes from the situation by hiding in a corner'. His life has become handicapped as a result in that he subsequently avoids socialising at parties despite invitations from friends, and works overtime in order to avoid attending political meetings in which he is very interested.

At assessment interview he was casually dressed, unshaven and avoided answering questions at times. His mood was low due to the problem he said, but he did not appear clinically depressed.

Mr Jones identified several key objectives and targets for treatment, which were: to be able to join a local social club and attend regularly for 3 hours twice a week; to be able to initiate and maintain a conversation with a woman of a similar age who is a stranger, for half an hour four times weekly; and, thirdly, to visit the local pub twice a week and engage and maintain a conversation for at least one hour.

Management of his problem will be on an out-patient basis and involve individual social-skills training using modelling and role-play, linked to graded exposure in real life to the anxiety-provoking situations. Regular intrasession practice will be given and clinical measures will be readministered 8 weeks after treatment starts.

In concluding strategies for cognitive behavioural assessment, it helps if you keep in mind your own objectives when planning and conducting an assessment interview.

Before you can plan your treatment programme, you will require a clear, objective and concise description of what the problems are, including what happens behaviourally, physiologically and cognitively to the client. You need to know when and where they occur, how frequently, and with what effect, emotion and consequence. This will include relevant history, but should focus mainly on the here and now. It should examine behavioural excesses and deficits and personal assets.

This information makes up your formulation, that is, the working hypothesis you use in identifying the nature of the problem. Formulations are made at various stages throughout therapy. The formulation made during the assessment phase will form the basis of future therapy. An accurate working hypothesis is an essential element of the assessment process.

To do this effectively, you will need to verify the client's verbal reports. This can be done by behavioural tests, interviews with relevant others and measurement (i.e. questionnaires). You will also have to identify the stimulus–response partnership, e.g. for spider fears:

- What kind of spider?
- What colour?
- How large?
- Moving or stationary?
- Tomato tops?
- Other insects?
- With what effect?

The client and therapist need common terms of reference, so the problem should be discussed, negotiated and agreed between them.

The assessment needs to place the client in his/her social and environmental context, examining and describing their marital and familiar relationships and background. Where relevant, detail sexual and social skills, relationships and difficulties; interests and employment should also be examined.

Previous treatment for psychiatric and physical problems needs to be examined as does any ongoing treatment, particularly medication and its effects.

The individual's motivation and self-control (desire to change, effects on others, evidence of change, reinforcers, etc.) needs to be described.

Assessment by describing difficulties and problems should lead you to being able to formulate targets and a plan of management, which will describe where you and the client are going, what methods and techniques you intend to use and some prediction of what results you intend within a specified time span.

To summarise:

What information have you at present?	**Data**	e.g. Referral letter, general practitioner's (GP) letter, social worker (SW) report
What more information and forms are required?	**Data**	e.g. Interview with client and relevant others
What do you make of what you've collected?	**Cognitive behaviour analysis & formulation**	e.g. List of problems, possible reinforcers
What are the first priorities for treatment?	**Targets**	e.g. Homework tasks
What ongoing measures are required?	**Data**	e.g. Record of homework, daily diaries, relaxation diaries
How will the problems be tackled?	**Techniques, strategies**	e.g. Use of home resources, use of co-therapists, education of relevant others

When things do not go as planned

Previous discussion in this chapter focused on the development of the therapeutic relationship and cognitive behavioural assessment. Unfortunately, however, there are occasions when interviews and relationships do not go according to prediction or as planned.

Before looking at the reasons why things don't always go as planned, it is useful to recall a general set of criteria that are commonly used broadly to assess client suitability for a cognitive behavioural intervention. It should be noted that criteria are flexible and are always changing, particularly in light of advances in therapeutic interventions.

Suitability criteria

1. The therapist and client agree to define the identified problem in terms of observable behaviour and reported cognitions.
2. The behaviour and cognitions can be understood in terms of a current and predictable pattern.
3. The therapist and client can agree on clear cognitive behavioural goals.
4. The client understands and agrees by informed decision to the type of treatment offered.
5. There are no contraindications to cognitive behaviour therapy (e.g. severe depression, active psychosis, organic dysfunction).

There is much written about why clients do not do well either at the assessment and formulation stage, or whilst in treatment. This part of the chapter will, however, focus on why things don't go as planned prior to a treatment programme starting.

Foa et al. (1983) for example, argue that, in the search for predictors of failure in treatment, it is only when investigation is carried out of the differences between those who succeed and those who fail, can light be thrown on the mechanisms involved in treatment and more effective treatment strategies be developed.

Unsuitability

The first point concerns the client who is not suitable for cognitive behavioural treatment. Clearly, psychotherapy is not for everybody and there are particular types of problems for which cognitive behavioural psychotherapy is not a treatment of choice.

Cognitive behavioural psychotherapy comprises a range of therapeutic strategies and interventions that aim to change abnormal behaviour and faulty thinking patterns directly as identified by the client, rather than by analysing hypothesised internal conflicts or past history. It has been used with several client populations, including children and adolescents, people with physical health problems, the elderly and people with learning disabilities. It is the treatment of choice for selected problems totalling about 15% of all psychiatric out-patients, although statistics vary according to different research reports, demographic variations and population densities.

Examples of types of problems unsuitable for cognitive behavioural intervention include severe depression, which hinders the effectiveness of treatment, active psychosis, for which cognitive behaviour therapy has had mixed outcomes both good and less positive, and organic dysfunction, in which there can be cognitive impairment and possible memory recall difficulties.

Refusal

Despite the therapist conducting a thorough and comprehensive cognitive behavioural assessment and formulating clear problem statements, the client may refuse to engage in treatment.

There are several reasons for this. The client may, after being in assessment for several sessions, realise that as soon as a treatment rational had been explained to them, they are capable of treating themself without the assistance of a therapist. In such a case, behavioural guidance and bibliotherapy can be used, as well as the offer of a follow-up appointment or telephone contact to provide the client with support in their endeavour to self-treat their problem.

Despite a clear outline of a treatment plan, the client may decide that the therapy is too hard for them to take on or that they are not as motivated to overcome their problem as they thought. It is not unusual for clients to want quick-fix solutions to complex problems, or expect the therapist to do most of the work to overcome the problem or the therapist to wave a magic wand that will change things instantly.

Clients have also been known to have been coerced into attending an assessment interview because the immediate family has had enough of the problem rather than the client wanting to overcome the problem him/herself. In these types of cases an in-depth assessment of motivation is clearly important. Behavioural tests are commonly used to discover the degree of commitment that the client is willing to give to treatment. An example of a behavioural test would be to ask a client with agoraphobia to demonstrate how far away from home they can walk alone without help, or to ask a person with an obsessive compulsive handwashing problem to shake hands with the therapist whose hand may be 'contaminated with germs'.

Another reason for refusal is that the treatment offered by the therapist is not what the client is seeking in terms of the type of intervention. As said before, cognitive behaviour therapy is not for everyone, the client may wish to engage in dynamic psychotherapy or counselling. It is appropriate in such a case to enable the client to achieve their goal of seeking therapy elsewhere by re-referring them on to a colleague, at least pointing them in the right direction to self-refer to another agency.

Therapist/client incompatibility

This aspect of when things don't go as planned is complex but several issues can be identified.

For whatever reason, the client and therapist may not get on together to form a positive working relationship. The construction of a solid working alliance is not always easy and some common areas for consideration include:

- Attitudinal issues, for example, the client may not wish to be interviewed by a therapist from an ethnic minority background or someone who has a particular regional accent.
- Gender is sometimes an issue and a female client may not like being interviewed by a male therapist, especially if the problem is of a sexual or marital nature. Aside from the usual issues of embarrassment, a female client may have been assaulted by a male, which makes the formation of a positive working relationship by a male therapist especially difficult.
- Age. It is not uncommon in the caring professions generally for clients to experience difficulty in relating to a person who is junior in years, and cognitive behaviour therapy is no exception to this. The youth of the therapist is sometimes a disadvantage in the eyes of the client who is looking for a worldly wise person to whom to disclose personal information.

- Socioeconomic factors are sometimes perceived by clients as an issue that hinders the development of a good therapeutic alliance. The therapist may be perceived as both educated and financially comfortable compared to the lot of the client. Clearly the cognitive set of the client can be, 'what does this therapist understand about my life and problems, they have a different existence to me'.
- Inexperience of the therapist is often an issue with the client who needs to have confidence and trust in the therapist, which is usually associated with the notions that the therapist knows what they are doing and are clinically competent to help them with their problem.

If it is the experience of the therapist that such factors are going to hinder the development of a good therapeutic relationship and the issues are unresolvable after detailed analysis, then it is appropriate to offer the client the option to receive cognitive behaviour therapy from a colleague, although there may be some practical problems of transferring clients between busy sectors or departments, or seek treatment elsewhere. This type of situation does not appear to happen too often in clinical practice and problem solving usually resolves most incompatibility difficulties.

Inappropriate strategy

The last issue of concern is the offering to the client of an inappropriate treatment strategy for a problem. This can be due to the inexperience of the therapist in terms of not having seen a particular problem previously, or not achieving a complete and functional analysis of a problem. Whatever the cause, the client's problem is not being managed effectively, which usually results in the client dropping out even before therapy starts.

The final section of this chapter looks at the notion of supervision and reflective practice in the context of assessment and formulation.

Supervision

Clinical supervision has been a feature of professional activity for people working in psychotherapy and counselling over at least the last 25 years. Clinical supervision as a concept, however, is difficult to tie down by definition, and it is commonly mistaken to be part of a management role or within the context of a mentorship, assessor or preceptor scheme.

The term 'supervisor' is often used to describe an interaction that is anything but therapeutic, bringing to mind the notions of unhelpful criticism, discipline and punishment. Supervision has also been perceived as an activity associated with an alien group of elitist practitioners whose clinical practice is far removed from the real world, thus becoming the prerogative of the few instead of meeting the needs of the many.

In the context of assessment and formulation in cognitive behaviour therapy, the act of clinical supervision in an ideal world is simply about giving T.L.C. to the supervisee:

■ **Trust** the supervisee to undertake the task of problem assessment and identification. We all make mistakes and have much to learn from them.
■ **Leeway** – giving the supervisee the space and freedom to act and complete the task without unnecessary interruptions.
■ **Contact** – talking to and touching the supervisee when appropriate, for example, during emotionally demanding occasions, it is helpful to place a hand on a shoulder to calm down and minimise the anxiety experienced by the supervisee.

In return for which the supervisor will receive:

■ **Truth** from the supervisee about how they are managing and coping with clinical practice.
■ **Loyalty** – the supervisee will be keen to engage in the process of clinical supervision and will be motivated to meet on a regular basis.
■ **Communication** – the supervisee is more likely to talk about his/her strengths, weaknesses, successes and aspects that s/he wishes to change within the assessment stage of therapy.

The process of clinical supervision

Clinical supervision can now be seen to be a process which is about joint ownership, rather than one person controlling and influencing another.

Whilst the model of supervision initially selected by the supervisor will depend on the school of counselling or psychotherapy to which they belong, whether it be behavioural, cognitive behavioural, humanistic, psychoanalytic or eclectic, the process of supervision can be understood in terms of a parallel process, which reflects that which occurs with a client in therapy.

The idea of giving trust, leeway and contact to a supervisee matches exactly the activities that are required to develop a therapeutic relationship and therapeutic alliance with a client, described earlier in this chapter. Similarly, receiving the truth, loyalty or commitment and communication are positive features that the therapist hopes to achieve with the client, in the same manner as the supervisor with the supervisee.

Methods of clinical supervision

The method and organisation of supervision is dependent on: the theoretical model used by the supervisor and the level of supervision required by the practitioner.

However, several methods of clinical supervision can be used:

- Live supervision in which the client, supervisor and therapist are in the same room.
- Live supervision in which the client and therapist are in the same room with an audio link to a supervisor, who observes through a one-way screen and gives feedback via an earphone that the therapist wears.
- Live supervision as above with the addition of a remotely controlled camera for recording and playing back at a later point.
- Recording sessions between a client and therapist using an audio tape and/or camera, which can be analysed later by the supervisor.

Clearly the method used in clinical supervision is also dependent on resources and facilities. Not all organisations have purpose-built units with one-way screens and remote cameras.

As well as the method, there are also several ways of organising clinical supervision.

Ideally, supervision during assessment, particularly for the trainee therapist, needs to be frequent and to consist of one to one sessions with an expert supervisor from his/her own professional discipline. The supervisor needs to have been orientated to the process of supervision and be aware of the commitment it requires in terms of time, style and outcomes.

If a supervisor from his/her own professional discipline is not available, then as a second option a supervisor from another allied profession can be sought. Although not ideal, the idea of multiprofessional supervision has been tried and tested with some success.

One to one peer supervision with people of a similar grade and expertise has also been used effectively to organise clinical supervision, as well as group supervision, which is shared across teams of professionals.

A group method of clinical supervision used is to develop a network of supervision for a group of people with similar expertise and interests who do not necessarily work together on a day-to-day basis.

In order to ensure that clinical supervision is meaningful to the supervisor and supervisee, it is important that good record-keeping of meetings is undertaken which should include discussion centred on the therapy sessions between the therapist and client, and the supervision sessions between the therapist and supervisor.

The format and style of record-keeping is a matter of personal choice, which should be needs led rather than organisationally driven. Examples include the keeping of a diary that records critical incidents, maintaining a portfolio, the use of a reflective practice journal and a log of problem-solving events and situations.

To summarise supervision:

- Clinical supervision takes time, effort and commitment from the supervisor and the person supervised.
- Clinical supervision does not fit easily into a diary full of appointments, meetings, courses and holidays.
- Plan ahead to ensure that supervision of clinical practice and case management fits naturally into everyday events.
- Clinical supervision should not be perceived as an irritant that can be taken off the agenda at the slightest small distraction.
- Supervisors and supervisees have limitations and imperfections.
- A supervisor is not all-seeing and all-knowing, is not omnipotent and omnipresent and does not possess deity-like qualities.
- Clinical supervision is a two-way learning process.
- As a supervisor, be prepared for thought-provoking and challenging material.
- Supervision helps to remind us of our human caring qualities.
- Supervision can be uncompromising in its clinical and intellectual rigor.
- It takes sensitivity and trust to be a good supervisor.
- Supervision, although hard work, is enjoyable and does give a sense of personal achievement and professional development.
- Decide earlier rather than later to develop a supervisor network for peer support.
- Supervision is not intrinsic to any one professional group, it can, however, be learnt.
- The qualified professional who thinks they know everything about themselves and their job should not be allowed the opportunity to hinder the progress of others in supervision.

The characteristics of supervision at the assessment stage of therapy are such that the supervisor needs to:

- Provide frequent and consistent clinical supervision and case management, which is a combination of live and recorded styles.
- Recognise the complexity of the assessment stage of therapy by ensuring regular hands-on and face-to-face contact with the therapist.
- Complete supervision documentation and return it promptly to the therapist.
- Identify therapist strengths and weaknesses as a clinician, particularly aspects of the therapeutic alliance, and discuss them.
- Discuss the personal and professional needs of the therapist.
- Integrate underpinning research into clinical practice.
- Act as a role model and facilitate graded experiences.
- Encourage therapist autonomy and maintain a professional attitude to the therapist.

Conclusions

This chapter has considered assessment and formulation in cognitive behaviour therapy, particularly the creation of the therapeutic relationship as a grounding for the therapeutic alliance in therapy. Three models of behavioural and cognitive assessment have been described in detail as well as the notions of unsuitability for therapy, and incompatibility between the therapist and client. Clinical supervision, concepts and processes conclude the chapter and draw together the themes within it.

There are several key issues from the chapter that are significant, and raise issues and implications for clinical practice.

Cognitive behaviour therapy is well established and grounded in empirical research over many years. The numbers of people practising as therapists with a professional qualification is rising steadily. In addition to which clinical supervision has now achieved a high place on the agenda. Whilst registration of psychotherapists in Britain and Europe is in its infancy, it is nevertheless of concern that cognitive behavioural psychotherapy is still being offered to clients by self-styled therapists without formal qualification and supervision. Clients are being assessed for cognitive behaviour therapy under false pretences of competency. Aside from the ethical, moral and legal dimensions of this issue, cognitive behaviour therapy, including assessment, can be complex and demanding, and it should never be undertaken by an unqualified practitioner who is not supervised. It is, therefore, the responsibility of the practitioner to ensure that s/he is fit for practice as a therapist by undertaking an appropriate qualification in cognitive behavioural psychotherapy and receiving regular clinical supervision.

Discussion questions

To what extent is the therapeutic relationship important in assessing clients problems?

What options are available to the therapist when the client refuses to attend for assessment interview?

How does an assessment model contribute to an understanding of a client's problem?

What qualities in a therapist are important for clinical practice?

References

Alexander, J.F., Barton, C., Schiavo, S. and Parsons, B.V. (1976) Systems-behavioral intervention with families of delinquents: therapist characteristics, family behavior and outcome. **Journal of Consulting and Clinical Psychology 44,** 656–664.

Bennun, I. and Schindler, L. (1988) Therapist and patient factors in the behavioral treatment of phobic patients. **British Journal of Clinical Psychology** 27, 145–150.

Cappella, J.N. and Street, R.L. Jnr. (1985) Introduction: A functional approach to the structure of communicative behavior. In Street, R.L. Jnr and Cappella, J.H. (eds) **Sequence and Pattern in Communicative Behavior**. London: Edward Arnold, pp. 1–29.

Curtis, J.M. (1982) The effect of therapist self-disclosure on patient's perceptions of empathy, competence and trust in analogue psychotherapeutic interaction. **Psychotherapy: Theory, Research and Practice** 19, 54–62.

Emmelkamp, P.M.G. and Van der Hout, A. (1983) Failure in treating agoraphobia. In Foa, E.B. and Emmelkamp, P.M.G. (eds) **Failures in Behavior Therapy**. New York: Wiley, pp. 58–81.

Foa, E.B., Steketee, G., Grayson, J.B. and Doppelt, H.G. (1983) Treatment of obsessive–compulsives: when do we fail. In Foa, E. and Emmelkamp, P.M.G. (eds) **Failures in Behavior Therapy**. New York: Wiley, pp. 10–34.

Ford, J. (1978) Therapeutic relationship in behavior therapy: an empirical analysis. **Journal of Consulting and Clinical Psychology** 46, 1302–1314.

Frank, J.D. (1982) Biofeedback and the placebo. **Biofeedback and Self-regulation** 7, 449–460.

Goldstein, A.P. and Myers, C.R. (1988) Relationship enhancement techniques. In Kanfer, F.H. and Goldstein, A.P. (eds) **Helping People Change**, 3rd edn. Oxford: Pergamon. pp. 19–65.

Hopkinson, K., Cox, A. and Rutter, M. (1981) Psychiatric interviewing techniques. III. Naturalistic study: eliciting feelings. **British Journal of Psychiatry** 138, 406–415.

Kanfer, F.H. and Saslow, G. (1969) Behavioral diagnosis. In Franks, C.M. (ed.) **Behavior Therapy: Appraisal and Status**. London: McGraw Hill, pp. 417–444.

Lang, P. (1970) Stimulus control, response control and desensitization. In Levis, D. (ed.) **Learning Approaches to Therapeutic Behaviour**. Chicago: Aldine Press, pp. 148–173.

Lazarus, A.A. (1973) Multimodal behavior therapy; treating the 'Basic Id'. **Journal of Nervous and Mental Disorders** 156, 404–411.

Morris, R.J. and Suckerman, K.R. (1974) Therapist warmth as a factor in automated densitization. **Journal of Consulting and Clinical Psychology** 42, 244–250.

Orlinsky, D.E. and Howard, K.I. (1978) The relation of process to outcome in psychotherapy. In Garfield, S.L. and Bergin, A.E. (eds) **Handbook of Psychotherapy and Behavior Change**. New York: Wiley, pp. 311–348.

Patterson, G.R. (1982) **A Social Learning Approach: Coercive Family Process**. Eugene, OR: Castalia.

Schaap, C., Bennun I., Schindler, L. and Hoogduin, K. (1993) **The Therapeutic Relationship in Behavioural Psychotherapy**. Chichester: Wiley, p. 3.

Schaap, C. and Schippers, G.M. (1986) Motivation strategies in the behavioral treatment of problem drinkers. **XVIth Annual Conference of the European Association for Behaviour Therapy**. Lausanne, Switzerland, September.

Schindler, L., Revenstorf, D., Hahlweg, K. and Brengleman, J.C. (1983) Therapist behaviour in behaviour therapy: Development of an instrument for rating by the client. **Partnerberatung** 20, 149–157.

Street, R.L. Jnr and Hopper, R. (1982) A model of speech style evaluation. In Ryan, E.B. and Giles, H. (eds) **Attitudes Towards Language Variation: Social and Applied Contexts**. London: Edward Arnold, pp. 175–188.

Tennen, H., Rohrbach, M., Press, S. and White, L. (1981) Reactance theory and therapeutic paradox; a compliance-defiance model. **Psychotherapy** 18, 14–21.

Truax, C.B. and Carkhuff, R.R. (1967) **Towards Effective Counseling and Psychotherapy**. Chicago: Aldine Press.

Further reading

Therapeutic relationships

Schaap, C., Bennun, A., Schindler, L. and Hoogduin, K. (1993) **The Therapeutic Relationship in Behavioural Psychotherapy**. Chichester: John Wiley and Sons.

Cognitive behavioural assessment

Bellack, A.S. and Hersen, H. (1988) **Behavioral Assessment**, 3rd edn. New York: Pergamon.

Failure in therapy

Foa, E. and Emmelkamp, P.M.G. (1988) **Failures in Behaviour Therapy**. New York: Wiley.

Clinical supervision

Hawkins, P. and Shohet, R. (1993) **Supervision in the Helping Professions**. Buckingham: Open University Press.

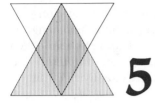 **5**

A Framework for Intervention

Andrew Stevens

Key issues

- The main phases common to most cognitive behaviour therapy interventions.
- The skills the therapist should pass on to the client.
- Some specific methods used to deal with specific difficulties.

Introduction/overview

Once the trainee therapist has absorbed the basic model, principles and 'textbook' methods of using a cognitive behavioural approach to helping people change, s/he encounters the 'real world' of assessment and formulation, and then the actual intervention. This chapter provides the therapist with a framework for intervention in a very practical way, describing the main phases common to most cognitive behaviour therapy (CBT) interventions and some of the pitfalls. It also prepares the ground for the important stages of generalisation and the client's maintenance of his/her newly acquired self-management skills – or relapse prevention, as this final step could otherwise be called.

Priorities for intervention

After the therapist has completed the assessment and formulation – or rather the provisional assessment and formulation, as both can change as more data about causational and maintaining factors come to light – then specific therapeutic steps can be derived. In deciding with the client what intervention is indicated, the following questions are usually relevant:

- What is the priority focus for intervention?
- In which area of possible intervention is change most likely to occur?
- Which 'vicious circles' are contributing most to the maintenance of the problem?

Some case studies

Throughout this chapter, four case studies will be used to exemplify some of the problems that specific clients present. These are listed below.

Client 1: a 40-year-old female, referred to as Liz, with severe and chronic depression. She has had a number of admissions to a psychiatric hospital. Her belief that she will ever 'get better' is very weak.

Client 2: a 22-year-old male, referred to as Don, with a recent onset of panic attacks. The thought 'I am going to go mad' is quite strong.

Client 3: a 32-year-old female, referred to as Ann, who self-mutilates and has low self-esteem, but for whom the intervention of choice is relationship therapy, if her partner will agree.

Client 4: a 22-year-old man with a learning difficulty, referred to as Tony, who has been excluded from his sheltered workshop placement because of aggressive behaviour towards a fellow worker.

The therapy contract

In general, agreeing a 'contract' with the client is a good idea. How specific this is will depend on aspects of the client's problem and possibly on some of the client's behaviour, in the case of clients who have been in therapy before – often on more than one occasion. Most contracts, however, will be quite simple and merely involve the number of sessions a client and a therapist agree to meet for before a formal review of progress.

Many of the classic well-controlled research trials of CBT methods have used in the order of 15–20 sessions. For many practising clinicians, a more likely number of sessions to choose is six or ten. The main advantages of stipulating the initial number of sessions is that the client knows what to expect, and the therapist can more clearly manage their workload. The disadvantages are for those clients who have a strong belief that they require an enormous amount of help before change is possible and who consequently do not commit themselves to a perceived 'inadequate' number of sessions. As long as the client comes back for the first session of this contract and does not pessimistically does not attend (DNA) at the first opportunity, this cognition can hopefully be dealt with in exactly the same manner as other more problem-bound cognitions.

Beliefs about therapeutic change

Some psychological attributes that may have a relationship to outcome in therapy are 'psychological mindedness' and 'readiness to change'. Work has also been carried out on the concept of 'pessimism', which may have an influence on both initial views of the likelihood of therapeutic change and future prevention (see, e.g. Seligman 1989). It is not usual to measure these formally in most routine therapy. Indications about the client's likely scores on such factors can usually be assessed by the sort of cognitions elicited in the course of the formulation interview. These concern the client's attributions about the cause of his/her problem and his/her beliefs about, specifically, the methods described by you, the current therapist, and, more generally, his/her beliefs about how human beings change – or, indeed, whether human beings **can** change.

Thus, a client who believes strongly that 'I am depressed because my father had the same problem, and depression is an illness transmitted genetically' is going to be fairly resistant to CBT methods for intervening with depression that focus on a learning model. Similarly, the client, who has a firmly held cognition 'for me to feel better, I shall have to say again and again to this nice therapist everything that has happened to me since the age of 5 years', will not be compliant with the type of sessions the enthusiastic cognitive behaviour therapist is planning.

Finally, some clients, especially when they have been involved in many previous completely or partially unsuccessful treatment methods, will have a very low level of therapeutic optimism and may even have rather egocentric beliefs such as 'well, these CBT methods may work for other people, but my problem is so severe/long-term, they are not going to work for me'.

Of course, all these thoughts are 'grist for the cognitive mill' and, if not dealt with, are likely to lead to both an even more despondent client, and a very frustrated therapist. These beliefs about therapeutic change cognitions can be conceptualised as the outer circle of a 'cognitive bull's-eye' (Figure 5.1).

The relationship between client and therapist

CBT requires a good relationship between therapist and client. Although other psychotherapeutic models put more overt emphasis on this relationship, factors such as the 'warmth, empathy and positive regard' of the

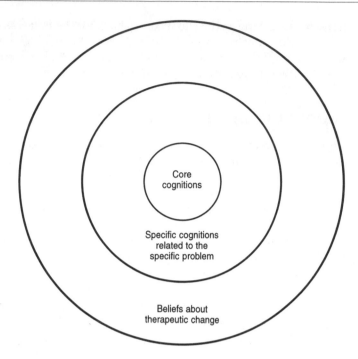

Figure 5.1　The cognitive 'bulls-eye'. A 'core' cognition is a deeply ingrained automatic way of thinking, often termed as 'schema' in cognitive therapy writings.

non-directive Rogerian school are important in CBT, as is the importance of a perceived 'collaborative effort' (e.g. Beck and Emery 1985: 173–176). Some of these non-specific components of psychotherapy can, of course, be 'translated' into cognitions, although it must be acknowledged that some might be 'unconscious' (i.e. the cognitions are ingrained and automatically assumed) to such an extent that they seem to be almost fundamental interpersonal processes.

It is important to be aware of the possible cognitive underpinning of such influences on the outcome of therapy. This is not merely cognitive pedantry, but lays the foundations for an analysis of various cognitive targets. This can be worked on in the early stages of therapy if it is clear to the therapist that one of these important interpersonal features is not evident in the relationship. Thus, a client who is saying to themselves 'this therapist just doesn't understand what I have been through' (that is, low perceived empathy) may well be quite resistant to taking anything the therapist says seriously. Note, however, that this low empathy thought itself may not be countertherapeutic in all cases. For example, a client who adds the subclause '... but that doesn't matter very much as I really need to learn how to get over what has happened to me', should be quite immune to the perceived lack of empathy.

Some clients may have cognitions about the therapist that are based much more on perceived competence than on the softer emotional components such as warmth and empathy. Although classical cognitive therapy is modelled on Socratic dialogue in which the therapist is the epitome of non-suggestion, in reality, many therapists find themselves drawn to provide pieces of information and to suggest to clients possible cognitions – either that they may be causational in their distress or ones they could use as antidote cognitions. Although it could be argued that the simple dominant aim of all CBT is for the client to learn how to best use the fundamental cognitive methods him/herself, there are situations when it is most cost-effective for the therapist to 'fill-in'. A client-led situation is when the client is so unused to monitoring his/her own thoughts or has learnt not to utter out loud their thoughts, that the therapist needs to offer multiple choices for what could be going on in the client's head. 'Is it possible that you are thinking ... or possibly ...?' One danger is, of course, suggestion, but this must be balanced against the frustrating scenario of the client repeatedly answering requests for cognitive self-monitoring with the ubiquitous 'I don't know'.

A therapist-led situation that condones the introduction of cognitions directly from the therapist is when the requirement to review a cognition leads to the need for the client to find out some more information. For example, a client with a fear of illness problem (often rather derogatively called 'hypochondria') may have a belief 'all breathlessness is a result of heart disease'. Now, the therapist may be sitting there knowing that some sensations of breathlessness in an individual can be caused by hyperventilation or shallow breathing (Salkovskis 1988). To inform the client of this fact – as long as the therapist is seen by the client as a (reasonably) 'high-status source', may be very anxiety reducing indeed. The client's fear of illness cognition is now modified to allow for 'breathlessness to be the result of a number of physical processes, some harmful and some benign. What is the probability that my current sensations are one or the other?'.

Strategies for intervening

Educating the client about the rationale behind the intervention is an important process. CBT involves the client learning some of the knowledge about psychological methods of change that initially reside with the therapist. Some psychotherapeutic approaches are much more concerned with the therapist somehow creating the conditions wherein the client will somehow change. For example, psychoanalytic therapists believe that making interpretations that provide the client with insight into their problem will allow change to occur. CBT is much more about the client making their own interpretations, once they understand the fundamental principles of the approach. CBT is a truly educational method. The cognitive behaviour therapist is in essence a teacher.

Therefore, in the early sessions of a CBT intervention, educating the client about both the basic principles and some specific methods or techniques deriving from the principles will dominate. In the session itself, the cognitive behaviour therapist may use diagrams on paper or on a convenient whiteboard. The use of cassette tapes – either prerecorded and standard, or recordings of the actual session itself, for the client to listen to between sessions – may well augment the educational content of the session.

'Selling' the rationale

Some mention of the need to influence the client's beliefs about the likely efficacy of a CBT approach has been described above in the section on 'Beliefs about therapeutic change'. This is not just relevant when the client is particularly cynical about the likelihood of achieving any change, but necessary with most clients. Some CBT ideas can sound deceptively simple. For example, saying to someone 'Well, once you have identified the problem thought, reviewed its accuracy and constructed an antidote thought, you just have to keep thinking it' could provoke the response 'If I could do that, I wouldn't need to be here in the first place!' So, the therapist needs to augment the message with some information about the notion of 'cognitive habit strength'. It takes a long time, and much persistent practice, to reduce the power significantly of an inaccurate and unhelpful thought that the client has had for many years. One additional component of a cognitive behaviour therapist's educational store is a collection of examples and anecdotes that illustrate various cognitive behavioural principles or techniques. These can be used to add reality to textbook descriptions and also to relate it to the client's own experience, if at all possible.

Use of literature and self-help books

As CBT is fundamentally an educational approach, it makes sense to use as many modalities to convey ideas as possible. Thus, written material is a common addition for the cognitive behaviour therapist. This can range from the single A4 leaflet, through the more substantial booklet to self-help books that are nowadays available from any medium-sized book-shop or even larger libraries. Reading to produce psychological change is, rather grandly, termed 'bibliotherapy'. Some research has been carried out into the efficacy of bibliotherapy (e.g. Scogin 1989). In general, the findings show that it is a useful addition to therapist intervention alone.

The content varies from a short description of a particular technique, such as how to plan a behavioural hierarchy in the case of a phobia, to full manuals for the cognitive behavioural treatment of depression or relationship problems.

The main problem facing most therapists who wish to use such material is the practical one of how to facilitate access to the material for a client. Whether to provide the material oneself or merely to give the client some titles of useful books is for each therapist to decide. The advantage of the therapist handing over the material directly to the client is that it is more likely to be read. The cost of this is of course greater and, unless the therapist has produced the material him/herself, there is also the legal issue of copyright, if the therapist plans merely to photocopy other people's self-help material.

Some therapists even give out articles from academic journals, either to reinforce some aspect of knowledge of the principles or possibly to help a client gain further information to review the accuracy of a particular thought. An example of this latter process might be for a client who had a strong belief 'there is no method available to treat my problem' to be given a paper showing that a group of people with a similar problem had indeed found a CBT treatment beneficial. Some clients who place great value on the empirical basis to the therapy that they are seeking out may be more influenced by such material than by rather more user-friendly, colloquial versions of the same theoretical and research material.

There is a problem using bibliotherapy routinely and frequently with some client groups, such as those with reading difficulties or a learning disability, and some children. However, as the cognitive behavioural principles and methods are the same for these groups, bibliotherapy material will be similar in content as for other client groups, but its preparation is likely to take more of the therapist's time. For example, a therapist could translate written material to audiotape for a client who cannot read well. Alternatively, educational material for a client with a learning disability could be restyled using much simpler language and illustrated as much as possible in diagrammatic form, for example, the use of cartoon drawings with 'speech balloons' may make both the concept and content of a cognition clearer to some clients. With Tony, a booklet on 'Managing your anger' seemed particularly appropriate, but as he could not read, this booklet was described to him in a joint session with his mother who would then be aware of the rationale and methods of a CB approach to anger management, and able to remind Tony about some of the techniques. Whenever relatives or others are involved in CBT, it is essential that the therapist prepares this person adequately. Some clients will perceive advice or reminders from a relative as 'nagging', which will probably be counterproductive. The best strategy is for the client to involve and brief the relative about his/her proposed role him/herself, so that the client retains full control.

General cognitive behavioural skills

The client needs to acquire some general skills – or at least improve on their prior level of skill – if s/he is to make the best use of CBT methods. These include:

- Increased self-awareness.
- 'Being one's own detective'.
- Persisting versus dabbling.
- Having an incremental, gradual view of change.
- Cures are not the aim.
- Planning.
- Measuring change.

In the following sections, each of these skills is discussed in turn concerning its nature and how it can help a client to develop.

Increased self-awareness

To be aware of one's thoughts is not straightforward. We all have thousands of thoughts every day. Many of these thoughts are not conscious. Many of our behaviours are under unconscious control, especially those that we have done so many times before; they have become habitual. It is highly likely that some of our emotions are also provoked by thoughts that are unconscious. If a client is going to be able to change some of their problematic behaviours and some of their unpleasant emotional experiences, s/he needs to be more successful at identifying the thoughts that are leading to these behaviours and emotions. Then, by reviewing and challenging these thoughts, the resulting behaviours and emotions will alter as well. This is the basis of cognitive therapy.

The thoughts that are related to actual situations or events in our lives can be termed 'object-related cognitions'. However, cognitive psychologists also use the term 'metacognition' to describe those thoughts, which are basically 'thoughts about thinking' (Wegner 1994). Thus, the thought 'that man who pushed in the queue really is very rude' would be an object-related thought that a person might have in response to a particular situation they found themselves in. However, 'the thought I've just had – about the man pushing in – is just the sort of thought I need to challenge if I'm going to control my anger problem' is a metacognition. Without the metacognition, the person will tend not to have any mechanism to review, and possibly challenge, his/her thinking. Therefore, to be good at self-awareness is another way of saying to be skilled in metacognition.

Because human beings are habit-ridden, it is important for a person who intends to use cognitive methods to slow down and turn their attention inwards to their thoughts more often than they usually do. To begin with, simple exercises can be suggested by the therapist. These need not be related to the problem itself. Indeed, it may be more productive for the client to try out an increase in self-awareness in very routine innocuous situations. If a client can become 'caught up' in the power of his/her own thinking early on in a therapeutic endeavour, then the prognosis is likely to be more favourable.

For example, the therapist can ask the client to analyse the process whereby s/he carries out an everyday activity. A common example, is learning to drive a car. Where do the thoughts come from that help a complete novice driver to actually turn right at a junction? The client can then be prompted to go through the following stages:

- Initially the thoughts come from the brain of the driving instructor.
- Then the driving instructor increasingly uses short phrases to indicate the same actions ('semaphore' language).
- Meanwhile, the pupil is beginning to say the instructions to themselves – often out loud initially.
- Gradually the instructor says less and less, unless a novel situation or crisis develops.
- The pupil then learns to have the thought running through their head quite briefly.
- Eventually, the pupil hardly thinks about driving at all whilst they are driving. His/her cognitive activity will be much more likely to be centred on what is on the radio, or what they are doing that evening, and so on.
- The pupil's driving behaviour is now under – largely unconscious – control.

Such an example can illustrate how even quite complex behavioural sequences and emotional states may become, via repetition and practice, under the control of particular cognitions. There is nothing mysterious about the process. One does not have to enter into a 5-year psychoanalysis to understand the likely basis of some initially quite odd behavioural and emotional disturbances found in human beings.

A second useful example is to focus the client on a behavioural sequence in which they have choices – rather than the complex visuo-motor task, such as driving a car – in which most choice is considerably limited due to the very overlearned and habitual nature of the task. Thus, for example, the therapist could ask the client why they eat what they do eat for breakfast. Most people do this every day, so the thoughts are usually not too difficult for them to access. Such mundane examples also allow those clients, who are not very proficient at, or are reticent about voicing their thoughts, a less threatening self-awareness exercise.

The thought sequence of one client proceeded as follows:

1. 'I usually eat some cereal and some toast.'
2. 'I suppose I usually eat an oat- or other fibre-based cereal because I think roughage is good for me.'
3. 'I would usually eat wholemeal toast for the same reason, although if I'm on holiday, or I'm feeling self-indulgent, I'll eat white toast with jam for a treat.'
4. 'I don't believe I have to be 100% the same in what I eat. Some variation is fine.'
5. 'I can remember my parents telling me that eating something substantial for breakfast was a good way to start the day'.

Even such a simple exercise can move from the simple cognitive level of describing the situation and how the person behaved in the situation, to the more complex (deeper) cognitions that underpin the behaviour. Thus, thought (2) above suggests the person may have a general relatively high self-esteem thought: 'I'm worth looking after'. Thoughts (3) and (4) show signs of a continuum way of thinking: 'Nothing is either all-black or all-white. Life is made up of different shades of grey'. Lastly, thought (5) shows the thinker beginning to analyse where some of the cognitions may have originated. The same can then be attempted for more clinically relevant behaviour and emotions.

Being your own 'detective'

Clients often say in answer to a question from their therapist 'I don't know'. This phrase can be heard in response to:

- Requests for descriptive information – when did something last occur and how often does it occur? and so on.
- Requests for cognitive information – what were you thinking at the time?
- Requests for formulation information – what could have caused you to feel that way?

'I don't know' is one of the most frustrating phrases a therapist can hear. However, most clients are bound to say it at some time or another. If a client knew all the answers, why are they seeing a therapist! But therapist and client need information to construct firstly a formulation, and then a management plan. Therefore, as a continuation of the assessment phase, it is important to cultivate in the client an enthusiasm for continuing to collect data – about behaviour, thoughts, emotions and physical states.

The assessment phase method of keeping a record of particular behaviours and cognitions can be continued throughout intervention. This step should remove some 'don't knows'. The continuing modelling of and encouragement to practice the 'Socratic method', which is a fundamental process in cognitive therapy, should reduce more 'don't knows', or at least force them to become 'I wonder why? Let me think about possible explanations'. Finally, if the 'don't knows' of a particular client are so frequent and habitual that their utterance seems to be hindering the whole session, the therapist can negotiate with the client whether they can agree either an 'allowance' or ration of 'don't knows' per session, or agree to a complete ban. As a further aid to the client, the therapist can offer to make some very obvious verbal or other behavioural sign (for example, putting a hand in the air as soon as the first syllables are spoken by the client) whenever the dreaded phrase occurs.

Persisting versus dabbling

Some clients seek help when they have very weak beliefs that they will ever be able to improve by their own efforts. The main reasons for this are listed below.

1. Someone else has been the impetus in making the clients seek help. For example, they are only attending for an appointment with a therapist because their doctor has told them to or perhaps they believe it will keep their spouse happy if they are 'seen to be doing something about their problem'.

2. They believe that if only they carry on seeking help, then one day, someone – other than themselves – will have the cure, the 'magic formula', the answer to their problems.

They find it more reinforcing to talk to someone else about their life and problems than actually doing something about changing themselves to enable the problems to reduce in size and become more manageable.

Eliciting these thoughts is as important a part of the assessment process as finding out about the presenting problem itself. These beliefs that suggest a low perceived possibility of therapeutic change will probably hamper any useful progress being made. They are very firmly on the outer circle of the 'therapeutic bull's-eye' described earlier in this chapter.

Of course, by their very either confidential or unconscious nature, they are not easy to elicit early on in therapy. A client, even if s/he has worked it out explicitly to him/herself will not like to admit to the therapist that 'I'm only here because my wife thinks I've got a problem' or 'my doctor has hinted they won't give me any more tranquillisers unless I come to see you'.

The cognition 'We meet together so I can tell you all about what's been happening to me in the last week, and that will make me feel better' is fairly common in some clients. This is the case especially when they have seen other therapists before who took a more cathartic or supportive stance than a cognitive behaviour therapist is likely to take. Thus, the client may have been reinforced by previous therapists that this is what the client role is, and is therefore what is expected of them.

Having an incremental, gradual view of change

It takes time to change ingrained psychological habits. Some clients take a very curative view and expect things to change quickly. Of course, some things can change quickly. A client who has very little hope – or a low degree of therapeutic optimism – can be influenced by the therapist saying something particularly hopeful and convincing. Thus, the statement by the therapist 'there's been a lot of research done that has shown that people with the type of problem you have can be almost completely recovered within 6 months' could lead to a significant improvement in mood in some clients. How accurate the therapist's cognition is that allows them to make this statement is, of course, another matter! Therefore, to look for some change in the first session and in subsequent sessions is quite appropriate. Indeed, if both client and therapist can see change occurring in all sorts of useful, albeit small ways, then they are both well attuned to the notion that psychological change is often gradual and incremental. However, for the client to experience a significant and substantial amount of change, to the extent that their original presenting problem is considerably improved, often does take time.

How much time will vary from problem to problem, and client to client. There are reports in the literature of, say, a monophobia, being almost completely deconditioned within 2–3 hours in one session. However, for many clients, progress will be over many weeks or even years. After all, surely we are all learning about life and the situations that could be handled differently all the time. This is an important perspective to have for all therapists – and their clients. If change does take years, does it mean the therapist has to continue seeing a client while all this change takes place? The answer is a clear 'no – only until the client has the psychological tools to make a better job of their life than they had been making prior to seeing the therapist'. It is important to clarify this early on in therapy, otherwise the client may have the implicit assumption that they have to remain in contact with the therapist until they have reached their final goal.

One way to illustrate this intended process of gradual change and finite contact with the therapist is to draw a diagram for the client, such as Figure 5.2.

Cures are not the aim

The task of discussing overtly with the client this notion of gradual change, involving trial and error, new learning, followed by practice and consolidation should help the client to have a much more constructive and long-standing view of what psychological therapy is all about. It is not about panaceas or being ephemerally influenced by the novelty of all the personal attention people in individual therapy receive. It is about

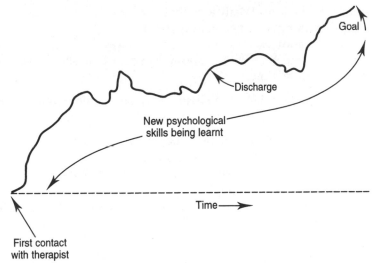

Goal

Discharge

New psychological
skills being learnt

Time ⟶

First contact
with therapist

Figure 5.2   An incremental, gradual view of change. The graph is not straight but 'bumpy' as trial and error have their influence.

hard and thoughtful work, the end result of which is not a 'cure'. It is a better rating on some of the key psychological skills that will enable a person to live a more satisfying and pleasurable life, and make it more likely that they will be able to solve problems that come their way – either external environmental problems or internal psychological ones.

Planning

Some clients do not need to plan how they are going to implement the CBT ideas they have learnt with the therapist – or from a book. It just seems that they can read, listen to and discuss some concepts and specific methods, and then go off and enact them. However, these clients are very definitely in the minority. Most people, when they seek to change some aspect of their behaviour or thoughts, will have to construct a plan, often quite detailed, and with a timetable, if they are to have any chance of achieving useful change.

The components of a CBT change plan usually consist of the 'what', 'when' and 'where' sections.

'What'

Which particular activities is the client going to do? For example, a behavioural 'what' could be:

- Keeping a written record of anxiety attacks.
- Going into a specific feared situation.

- Planning a schedule of daily activities.
- Saying something to someone in particular.
- Doing a relaxation exercise with a cassette tape.
- Setting up a meeting with a specific person that should last for a certain amount of time.

It is as important to help the client focus on cognitive aims as well. Examples could be:

- Trying to 'catch' thoughts that the client has when in a specific situation or mood state – and write them down.
- Constructing an antidote thought to be used to challenge a particularly frequent problem thought.
- Stopping a certain thought that the client finds especially repetitive and disturbing.

'When'

When are the 'what's' going to be carried out? For example, the 'when' could be:

- Every day, until the next therapist/client session.
- Twice a day, once before breakfast, and once in the early evening.
- For a 3-hour period every morning.
- Every time the client finds him/herself in a particular situation.
- Four times before the next session.

'Where'

Where are the 'what's' planned to happen? For example:

- At home.
- At work.
- In specific shops of a particular type or size.
- In a cafe or pub where the client will not be interrupted by family members.

Notice how the words 'specific', 'particular' and 'certain' keep appearing in the above examples. The specifying of the behaviours, how often it should be attempted and the location are not just pedantic, overcontrolling therapist tendencies. Behavioural change is more likely to occur if it is well-defined or 'concrete' (rather than vague) and attempted in small, manageable steps. However, remember that the therapist does not want to have to take each small aim and help construct a plan for it. Rather, the therapeutic goal is to focus on the clients themselves acquiring the skill of planning in general, so the therapist can concentrate on the overall direction or strategy, as well as helping solve particular problems that occur.

Measuring change

The measurement of personal change is a component of successful CBT. If a person makes efforts, it is important that s/he has a mechanism that tells him/her 'you are doing well, keep at it'. Otherwise, premature discontinuation of methods that would otherwise result in substantial benefit to the person can occur. Some measurement possibilities will have arisen out of the assessment stage of CBT. These can provide an overall perspective on the amount of change achieved since the client first presented for help.

However, the planning process described above will also suggest many opportunities for assessing progress. This is a spin-off from the principle of defining aims within the plan in a specific and detailed manner. It is usually clear to both client and therapist whether such aims have been achieved, and thus progress is being made. (Do note, however, that a client can carry out all aspects of an agreed plan between sessions and still report that no progress is being made! This could be due to the client expecting very quick and large change, or because some of the tasks s/he carried out did not have the consequences that both client and therapist thought they were likely to have. If the latter occurs, then the progress to be made is in the increased understanding that follows this real data feeding back into the overall formulation and plan of action, and the client reperceiving the actual carrying out of the tasks as the success, albeit if only a partial one).

Problems in measuring change are much more likely to come about when the aims are described in a very general, global manner. This is more of a fundamental problem for psychotherapeutic approaches other than CBT.

Reviewing a thought

Once a client is aware of a thought that seems to be related to their presenting problem, they need to be able to review the thought: to take a look at it in a measured and structured manner. The first step of this review is to basically ask themselves 'is this thought accurate?' Other ways to ask this question are 'what is the evidence for this thought?' 'how true is it?'. The three usual ways to do this are given below.

1. The thought is assessed against the client's own experience. Often, even using their own experience alone shows many clients that the thought they were thinking – and perhaps very commonly and with a good deal of strength – is not accurate. Thus, for example, Liz would have the frequent cognition 'The best thing to do when I feel this depressed is to go to bed'. However, when prompted to ask herself how accurate this thought was, that is, 'has this strategy worked in the past?', she could

think of many times when going to bed had either made no difference, or indeed made her feel even more depressed.

2. Obtaining information from elsewhere is another method to review the accuracy of a thought. Thus Don used to think 'My panic attacks mean that I am going to go mad and end up in a psychiatric hospital'. He could not generate any evidence from his own experience to counter this thought. He had never known anyone who had had such apparently overwhelming physical sensations, nor had he had enough panics himself to realise that, very unpleasant though they were, he would recover. However, by setting himself the task of finding out more information by reading about panic attacks, he was able to see that panic attacks were indeed quite common phenomena, and were explicable by a rather different psychophysiological mechanism than 'going mad'.

3. Carrying out a behavioural experiment – or to 'reality test' – is a third, often very powerful, method to review the accuracy of a thought. Thus Ann identified the thought 'I cannot say anything at a parents' meeting at my child's school, as I am bound to forget what I am talking about half way through'. This thought had led to her always staying silent in this type of social situation, and thus she had no evidence from her own experience to challenge the thought. Nor was it easy for her to seek out information elsewhere to challenge the thought. Therefore, it seemed to her that the simplest method to review the truth of the thought was to actually say something in a meeting.

These types of review methods are often made clearer if the initial thought is written down using the double-column method. The three examples above would be written as follows:

Problem thought	Challenge or antidote thought
When I feel this bad the best thing to do is to go to bed.	When I feel this bad, going to bed has helped sometimes, but I often feel worse afterwards, and therefore I will probably be better off if I make myself do something physical – to see if it helps.
My panic attacks are so frightening, I'll end up going mad and be put in a psychiatric hospital.	My panic attacks are very unpleasant but I know that many do have panic attacks, and that they are a sign of stress, not madness. I focus on ending up in a hospital because that's what happened to my mother, but she had a postnatal breakdown.
I cannot say anything at a parents' meeting as I am bound to forget what I am talking about.	I do get anxious about making a fool of myself, but many of the things other people say are not that impressive. If I plan a likely comment beforehand, keep it short and write it down, then the odds are it'll come out OK, and I must get started somewhere to overcome my fear.

Notice how the antidote thought is considerably longer than the problem thought. This is quite usual. The problem thought is often a shortish 'personal cliché' that the client has thought many times before, and which has so often gone unchallenged that the person has an automatic and unquestioned belief in its accuracy. The antidote cognition will be longer because it is really a balanced and logical attempt to debate the key 'facts' in the problem thought.

Probability as a central concern

In the examples above of problem thoughts, the words 'best', 'end up' and 'bound to' are all categorised by their absolute nature. They are words that suggest the person is assuming that there is only one possible outcome that could occur. The person cannot apparently conceive of there being any other likely outcome, and therefore has not developed any alternatives or options. This is a common feature of problem thoughts, and is concerned with the probability of an event or a certain outcome occurring. Reviewing the probability element in a thought is typically one of the clearest and often strongest ways to help a client challenge that thought. Thus, in the first example above, the word 'best' suggests that, at the time of deciding what to do when feeling tired and depressed, Liz was only aware of that one thought. There was no distinct metacognitive process occurring, such as Liz thinking 'Wait a minute. This is one of my typical depressive thoughts. Are there any other thoughts I could be generating about this situation I find myself in?'

Another way of presenting this issue of choice amongst a number of possible cognitions to a client is to describe a 'thought pie'. The therapist can draw a circle and split it up into sections as in Figure 5.3a.

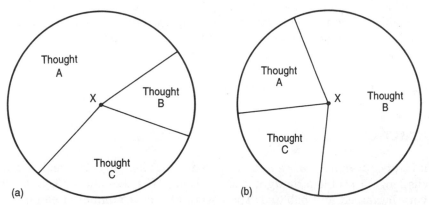

Figure 5.3 (a) and (b)   'Thought pies' to illustrate choice in thinking.

The person can then perhaps visualise more clearly that at point X, there are in fact a number of possible thoughts to have. The dominant one will usually be the one that is strongest in habitual terms – the one s/he has thought most often in the past without challenge. However, the others exist, and once the client can clearly see they exist, even though they are less powerful, then by repeated reviews and debate about the accuracy of each, the size of the piece of pie corresponding to each cognition can alter. Thus, after some time, self-awareness and practice, the above pie might have changed to the one shown in Figure 5.3b.

The helpfulness of a thought

Of course, many cognitions that a client reviews will appear to be very accurate, even after repeated analysis. For example, in someone who has failed an exam 12 times already, the day before they are sitting the exam for the 13th time, the thought 'it is highly likely that I shall fail tomorrow' may well be rather accurate. However, what is the effect of thinking this way? If passing is still very important to the person, s/he may become very anxious and this anxiety may well lead them to perform even less well than s/he otherwise would have, due to effects of anxiety on recall of information and so on. Alternatively, the cognition may lead them to abandon all hope of passing and not do any more revision at all. Who knows? Perhaps a few more hours of revision would have provided them with material to answer that vital surprise question? Thus, although the thought seems accurate, it could not be said to be a particularly helpful thought. Therefore, it can be challenged on that basis and a more helpful thought constructed as an antidote.

For example, Liz's evidence told her that going to bed did sometimes make her feel better. There was evidence from her own experience that sometimes a sleep did genuinely refresh her but, if she forced herself to look at how many times a sleep actually helped, she realised it was probably only one time in every five. Thus, the probability was 20%, and yet her assumption when she felt like going to bed was – relatively unconsciously – more like a 100% prediction of benefit. Therefore, although the thought 'sometimes a sleep will help' was accurate, for four out of five times, it was not helpful.

Practice

It is, of course, not sufficient merely to ask the client to catch, review and challenge a problem thought once or twice. The thought is likely to be very ingrained and habitual. There may also be a number of emotional associations with some thoughts that make them very difficult to handle in a more accurate or helpful manner. The client will usually need to practise thinking the antidote thought in situations when s/he used to think the problem thought hundreds of times, if the new thought is to become at all regular. It takes even more practice to make the alternative more productive cognition the habitual one. This gradual process must be clearly described to the client, otherwise, when the old cognition appears in all its vivid strength, the person may say to him/herself 'this cognitive therapy really doesn't work' and then stop using the method very prematurely. A more accurate – and helpful – cognition for him/her to have would be 'This cognitive therapy will take a lot of repeated and persistent effort. I must give the method a chance to cause me to feel better – or even a lot better – by challenging the thoughts that make me feel bad again and again . . . and again, and again and again . . . '.

There are exceptions to this rather incremental view of cognitive change. Sometimes a thought does change in an abrupt way and then stays that way without the person having to challenge the old thought repeatedly. The reader can probably think of some examples when this has happened to him/herself. For instance, you may have had a relationship of a certain type with a person that led you to always think about that person in a particular way. Then, one day, that person behaved in a manner that caused you to change that thought, and you subsequently found that you always thought about that person in the new way. This type of one-trial learning is not uncommon in everyday life and seems to be more often a result of a real-world experience rather than purely a consequence of internal cognitive activity.

Another occasion when a quick cognitive change occurs is when a person finds out a factual item of information that casts significant doubt for him/her on a belief s/he might have held up strongly until that point. For example, a person who previously believed that a type of food was completely health-giving could well change that thought if s/he read an article in a magazine, which reports that this food was linked to cancer in a whole series of laboratory experiments on mice. This sort of 'visionary' cognitive change happens frequently, of course, in everyday life but does seem to be less common in clinical work, where persistent and patient endeavour is required to effect change.

Specific methods for specific problems

The general cognitive methods described above are, for many clients, not only the most important skills at which they need to become fluent in order to bring change to their emotional state, but for some clients probably the only methods required to do this. However, some problems that clients present with do require specific additional methods, which will usually be behavioural. The commonest of these are:

- Exposure for phobias, obsessional and some other problems.
- Contracting and communication skills for relationship problems.
- Time management and activity scheduling for stress problems and depression.

Exposure methods

The behavioural method of exposure has a well-researched history as a fundamental technique in a cognitive behavioural approach. The classical problem area for which exposure is indicated is that of phobias. Exposure involves the person entering a situation that causes them anxiety and not escaping from that situation. As long as the situation is not one associated with any real threat to the person, then the anxiety will diminish even with the person staying in the situation. This may take some time but some phobias have been treated in this way in a matter of hours. Of course, many clients will hear about this exposure method and presumably never return to that therapist again as the technique sounds particularly unpleasant. Therefore an integral part of using the method is for the therapist to describe in detail the following points.

1. The 'extinction curve'. This is a visual description of what happens to the most unpleasant feelings of anxiety – as long as the person does not escape. This curve is shown in Figure 5.4. This diagram is worth drawing out during the verbal explanation as it conveys very clearly some 'light at the end of the tunnel'.

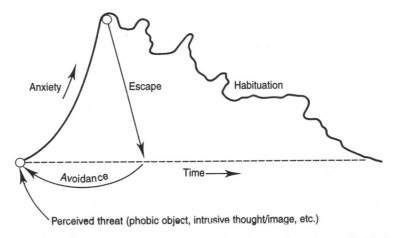

Figure 5.4   The extinction curve. For a phobic, escape and subsequent avoidance – if possible – manage the anxiety for a while, but only by going through the habituation curve can the anxiety be truly deconditioned.

2. A gradual approach is the method of choice. This means that the client is not usually advised that they should go into their most feared situation immediately, but that they should draw up a hierarchy or 'ladder' of feared situations, from easiest to hardest. They should then plan an approach to the first and easiest situation, and learn to cope with that one before moving on to the next stage on the hierarchy. An example of a hierarchy for Don was as follows:

Most difficult

↑ Driving alone for 100 miles on a motorway.

Driving alone on a motorway.

Driving 10 miles alone on a dual carriageway.

Driving with someone on a motorway.

Driving with someone on a busy A road.

Going on a road with roadworks.

↓ Stopping at traffic lights.

Easiest

3. The need to practice should be emphasised to the client. As with cognitive change, habits require considerable and repeated challenges. The same is true for ingrained behaviour patterns and certainly the highly conditioned emotional reactions associated with phobias. How much practice depends on a number of factors, but the inexperienced therapist can, unfortunately, create the wrong expectations in a client by implying that one or two exposure episodes will dramatically decondition strong psychophysiological reactions to particular situations.

A good example is with, say, an agoraphobic problem when the client may absorb the general principle of the exposure and habituation technique, and then proceed to seek out practice in their particular situation once or twice a week for 20–30 minutes. In fact, although there is a great range in the time required, an agoraphobic client may well need to spend hundreds of hours over a period of months in feared situations before they experience any appreciable and lasting improvement. Certainly there is evidence that 'massed practice' – longer practice sessions over a limited period – is superior to 'spaced practice' – shorter sessions (even if there are more in total) spread out over a longer period (Stern and Marks 1973). However, the theory of optimum exposure must be balanced against the wishes and practical circumstances of any specific client. The therapist should remember that it is their job to describe the methods and principles of CBT; it is up to the client to decide to implement any of the methods and how much effort to contribute.

The present chapter is only designed to provide a framework for intervention. There are other books that describe, in considerably more detail, methods such as the exposure technique for the deconditioning or desensitising of a phobia (e.g. Butler 1989). Before using these specific methods with clients, the therapist would be well advised to consult with such 'manuals' for further details of particular behavioural methods.

Exposure techniques are also pertinent to any type of problem in which the client usually tends to avoid or escape from a situation rather than go into or stay in it. Obsessional problems have the clearest parallel to phobias, except that the phobic object for the obsessional is one that cannot be avoided as it is so common in the person's external environment (dirt, germs, etc.) or it is internal, that is, a thought that is triggered frequently (e.g. the possibility of something going wrong, such as someone coming to harm, or the person him/herself losing control). Exposure techniques for obsessional problems are very similar to those for phobic problems, but other jargon such as 'response prevention' to describe the stage of non-escape are often used in behavioural literature.

Skills development through exposure

Exposure techniques are also relevant when a person cannot be said to be phobic of a situation, but has developed a habit of avoidance because they do not believe that they have the skills to achieve success in those situations. An example would be when a person has a social skills deficit. Thus, for Ann, who had quite low self-esteem, a self-managed programme of gradually facing more and more challenging social situations was seen as essential, if she was to undermine some of the antecedent conditions that made her more vulnerable to the risk of self-harm whenever she experienced even minor rejections by her partner. Ann developed a hierarchy similar to that of a phobic person, and then had to work hard at seeking out – or even developing from scratch – opportunities to engage in a novel and sometimes quite exploratory level of conversational skills.

Emotional processing through exposure

The term 'emotional processing' describes the mechanism whereby a very intense emotion is elicited in a person, usually repeatedly, causing the emotion to become 'processed'. That is, the emotion lessens in intensity, and is gradually assimilated into the person's world view at a physiological, behavioural and cognitive level.

This process is similar to that of desensitisation in phobias, but it is the intensity and the despair of the emotion concerned that is different in scale in emotional processing. Examples of this technique's appropriate use is in problems of post-traumatic stress disorder or in abnormal bereavement reactions. By not avoiding the stimuli that are associated with the intense emotion – for example, revisiting the scene of the incident or photographs of the deceased – and then not 'escaping' from the ensuing emotion, as the person perhaps previously did by, say, distraction techniques, the emotion can take its 'natural' course and abate in strength.

This example provides an interesting aside on the question clients often ask 'when should I distract myself from a problem thought and when should I confront it?' Although each situation should be judged on its own merits, a general guiding principle is as follows:

- Confront – that is, review the evidence for a cognition, and attempt to construct an antidote cognition – when little or no effort has yet been expended on that particular thought.
- Distract – or thought-stop – when considerable attention has already been focused on reviewing and challenging a particular cognition. If a thought is still causing a problem following substantial analysis and challenge, then it is likely that it is the habitual nature of the cognition that is problematic. To continue going through the whole review and challenge process each time the thought occurs is in fact likely to be mere rumination and may well be reinforcing the thought not weakening it. In such cases, distraction or thought-stopping are highly indicated.

Thus, exposure can be seen to be a broad-spectrum cognitive behavioural method, which forms one of the most useful techniques within a cognitive behavioural framework for intervention.

Contracting and communication skills

Many presenting problems, whatever the clinical diagnosis, such as depression, anger management or psychosexual disorders, are fundamentally often about the client's difficulties in developing or maintaining satisfying relationships. Therefore, if the formulation of the client's problem involves features, such as marital conflict, poor assertion skills and so on, the two skill areas of communication and contracting are likely to be components of the advised intervention.

Communication deficits are ubiquitous in human relationships. People either are not articulate or brave enough to say what they think, or one or more, usually both members of a relationship, have developed very powerful methods to deter the other from making the open and expressive comments that are surely the bedrock of most satisfying relationships. Once again, it must be pointed out that this chapter is not intended to supply a full account of communication skills teaching and the reader is strongly advised to obtain more dedicated accounts of CBT approaches to relationship problems, e.g. Schmaling et al. (1989). However, the following techniques do provide a framework for this skills area.

Often the first stage in improving communication in a relationship is for the participants in that relationship to agree to put specific time aside to talk to each other. This may sound rather obvious! However, it is typical in relationship problems that the parties do not do this, either because they have lost the habit of spending time on the relationship or emotional conflict has led to them avoiding such situations as they have been experienced as aversive. Thus, advice to spend a minimum of, say, one hour on an initially quite frequent basis talking to each other is a usual first step. Do remember that even this apparently simple manoeuvre is certainly not so simple for some couples. They will agree wholeheartedly in the therapy session that they will do this and yet return having avoided face to face communication. It may be necessary to advise that the parties actually set a fixed 'appointment time', otherwise the old habit of mutual avoidance will dominate.

During this communication period, it may become evident that one party is doing all the talking. This may be what typically happens during their relationship anyway. Of course, if the couple find this effective, then so be it but, in general, it is more productive if all parties have an opportunity to express themselves. To achieve this, the therapist can provide advice on an option for structuring the communication session, which has been called co-counselling. This involves the participants taking turns to be speaker and then listener, and splitting the available time approximately equally between them.

It is not always necessary – or most effective – for the parties to have only face to face communication. Writing to each other may be a useful method, especially when one of the relationship finds a physical presence inhibiting. Thus, Ann found that she was able to express herself much more clearly through writing to her partner than in actual meetings, partly because she was so habitually unassertive that, even when she had a clearly sanctioned opportunity to talk, she found it difficult, and partly because she was 'naturally' quiet, whereas her partner was talkative whatever the setting.

Once the parties are organising a structure for communication, they may still require some modification in how they express themselves. For example, one member of the relationship may routinely start any session with a list of criticisms of the other. This may disrupt the session as the target of this criticism becomes so angry, s/he leaves or fights back in a manner that further 'closes down' the open communication channels.

The skill of contracting can provide further guidance about the content of the more open communicative process. Contracting is a behavioural technique that has been used since the earliest days of behavioural approaches to marital dysfunction (Stuart 1969). The essence of contracting is for the parties to each state 'I would like X to happen, and if you do X, I am willing to do Y, which I believe you would like me to do'. Of course, it helps if the activities X and Y are approximately balanced in some way, but both parties usually have to accept that this is not always possible. Some give and take needs to occur.

It is also important that X and Y are explicitly defined, and not left as vague requests that are difficult to quantify. Otherwise, there will be disagreement about whether the other has fulfilled their side of the contract, even when each maintains that they have! It is essential that the members of the relationship take time to review the state of any contract they have set up. Contracting, like any other cognitive behavioural method is a skill that requires repeated practice, and an acceptance that some trial and error learning is unavoidable.

Although the commonest relationship that requires some attention in any psychological therapy is one involving two people, the communication and contracting approach can be used with families and employee/boss relationships. It can also be used by the presenting client unilaterally when either their partner cannot become directly involved in the therapeutic situation themselves, or when it is merely inappropriate for them to become involved.

An example of this latter situation was when Liz was cognitively 'catastrophising' about a planned visit to her partner's mother. She was anticipating that this lady would say a number of disparaging things about 'people with psychiatric problems', as she had always done in the past. Of course, Liz could have attempted to alter her own cognitions in a number of ways to reduce her emotional distress in this situation, but she decided to try a contracting option in which, at the beginning of the visit, she would ask her mother-in-law if the two of them could have a discussion about 'people with psychiatric problems' for a set amount of time. Liz would agree to listen and partake in the discussion but requested that there would be no mention of the issue outside this time.

This would obviously lead to a very artificial situation. However, the hallmark of the cognitive behaviour therapist as scientist–practitioner is to believe 'if it works (without deleterious side-effects), do it'.

Time management and activity scheduling

The skill of structuring how a person organises their activities into the time available is fundamental to many cognitive behavioural approaches and is, indeed, a broad-spectrum competence. One of the commonest occurrences is in CBT for depression where an increase in the amount of activity is seen as fundamental, if the client is to even have the possibility of augmenting the rewards they obtain from life. Authors such as Aaron Beck (1979) have described such techniques in detail in the form of a 'structured activity schedule' wherein the person rates the amount of mastery or achievement and pleasure experienced during each activity. For clients with a lot of vegetative symptoms, this behavioural stage of a managing depression programme is often essential before a cognitive emphasis can be assimilated.

This may seem paradoxical but a similar analysis of activities and timetabling is also indicated when a client is apparently doing – or attempting to do – far too much in their daily routine. Such behaviour will typically present as a stress problem and some improved time-management skills are called for. Once again, there are comprehensive manuals available that describe the therapeutic nuances of such approaches (e.g. Fontana 1993) and the reader is advised to consult such literature.

When early success is elusive, or when things do not go to plan

The framework described above should provide most therapists with a structure for intervention. A fundamental grasp of both the simplicity and the sophistication of a cognitive model is essential for effective therapy, and the three very broadly applicable specific methods will augment a cognitive outlook and derived techniques. It is worth emphasising at this point that very rarely does a therapist advise a client of the option of using a purely behavioural technique. There are almost always cognitive aspects to behavioural methods. Likewise, a behavioural component is often implied in the application of a cognitive stage of therapy.

One of the strengths of CBT is that the therapist should always have some ideas about what to do next! This applies equally well to both the first postformulation intervention, and the cultivation of possible options when progress seems to be either slow or absent. A check-list for action in the latter circumstance is given below.

1. Reformulate the problem. Has new information come to light during the first attempt at applying CBT that indicates some of the factors are either more complex, or have a different relationship to each other than was first thought?

2. Would it be worth going back a stage? For example, in a phobic problem, a strategic retreat to an earlier step on a hierarchy to consolidate at that level may be indicated.

3. Are there any aids that could be added to increase the rate of progress? For example, is some medication indicated or would the addition of a co-therapist, such as a partner or friend, be possible?

For example, Tony – with a therapist – generated a number of cognitions to act as self-statements that would maintain his awareness of the need for him not to become aggressive at his workplace. To help him make these thoughts more automatic and habitual, his therapist (with Tony) made an audiotape of them, which he agreed to play each day before he went to work. However, it became clear that he was forgetting to do this regularly, and therefore he was asked if he would consider involving his mother as a co-therapist. This suggestion worked well and led to involving his manager at work as well in planning with Tony a well-rehearsed 'escape routine' if he felt himself to be getting potentially aggressive.

4. Has the therapist been complacent about the client's knowledge of the cognitive behavioural approach – whereas, in fact, there are core gaps that are undermining the client's ability to use the methods effectively or generate the required degree of persistence? One way to find out is to test (diplomatically) the client's cognitive behavioural knowledge – asking them what they would advise a friend to do with a similar problem, not providing a ready answer during the therapy session. This latter is very difficult for some therapists, especially with quiet or slow-speaking clients, but even the most garrulous therapist can learn to programme themselves not to say something.

5. Scan for 'blocking cognitions'. Often these are on the outer circle of the 'cognitive bull's-eye' described above, and often they remain unuttered for long tracts of therapy time. Yet it is these that are impeding progress. 'If I get better, you'll discharge me, and I do so like coming' and 'I still think the problem is physical, and if only someone would give me the right test, everything would be alright' are but two, not so uncommon examples.

Supervision

One aspect of CBT is that it is relatively easy for people with even a small amount of theoretical and practical knowledge to think they know how to intervene with a client's problem. The advantage of this is that the ideas and methods can spread and be utilised without potential therapists having to spend years on time-consuming and esoteric courses. However, the disadvantage of CBT being apparently so straightforward is that clients can be poorly advised by inexperienced therapists who have grasped the basic principles and the outline of a few core techniques. These techniques are then used in rather a 'cook-book' fashion with very little flexibility of application whatever the needs of a particular client.

Such a scenario can lead to disillusionment on the part of both client and therapist. The client will not experience the benefit they were expecting, lose any confidence they had in a CBT approach, and retreat at a very premature stage to their prior method of coping, or move on to another type of therapy. The therapist who is both inexperienced and basically very generic in orientation, owing to their mixed and rather superficial training in a number of varied psychotherapeutic approaches, will likewise – at a premature point in therapy – begin to experience cognitions such as 'perhaps the problem does lie in this client's child-hood?' The answer from a therapist who has a more coherent and comprehensive view of CBT is 'of course, this client's experiences in childhood are the – at least partial – cause of the problem. Where else would they have begun to learn to think the sort of thoughts they now experience as very ingrained habits?'

So, despite the apparent simplicity of the principles of CBT, the practice requires of the therapist continuous self-appraisal, and subsequent modification of content and therapist style. Supervision by a more experienced colleague is essential, but the supervisee should be vigilant. S/he should choose a supervisor who really is competent in their grasp of the depth and sophistication of a cognitive and behavioural approach to helping humans in distress, or s/he will have much narrow thinking and frustration to experience.

Discussion questions

(A) This chapter describes cognitive behaviour therapy as a truly educational method which may make use of literature and self-help books. How can this 'bibliotherapy' be accommodated when the client is a child, a person with a learning disability or someone whose first language is not English?
(B) Cognitions about the process of therapy are described as important in this chapter. When the cognitions are negative but unrelated to the referred problem, is it reasonable to spend time in addressing these unrelated cognitions?
(C) The techniques described in this chapter could seem to offer a panacea for all ills. What features of the client or their presenting problem would indicate that cognitive behaviour therapy would not be the appropriate intervention to use with them?

References

Beck, A.T. and Emery, G. (1985) **Anxiety Disorders and Phobias: A Cognitive Perspective**. New York: Basic Books Inc.

Beck, A.T., Rush, A.T., Shaw, B.F. and Emery, G. (1979) **Cognitive Therapy of Depression**. New York: Guildford Press.

Butler, G. (1989) Phobic disorders. In Hawton, K., Salkovskis, P.M. et al. (eds) **Cognitive Behaviour Therapy for Psychiatric Problems: A Practical Guide** pp. 97–128. Oxford: Oxford University Press.

Fontana, D. (1993) **Managing Time**. Leicester: British Psychological Society.

Salkovskis, M.P. (1988) Hyperventilation and anxiety. **Current Opinion in Psychiatry** 1, 76–82.

Schmaling, K.B., Fruzzettii, A.E. et al. (1989) Marital problems. In Hawton, K., Salkovskis, P.M. et al. (eds) **Cognitive Behaviour Therapy for Psychiatric Problems: A Practical Guide** pp. 339–369. Oxford: Oxford University Press.

Scogin, F., Jameson, C. and Gochneaur, K. (1989) Comparative efficacy of cognitive and behavioural bibliotherapy for mildly and moderately depressed older adults. **Journal of Consulting and Clinical Psychology** 3, 403–407.

Seligman, M.E.P. (1989) Explanatory style: predicting depression, achievement and health. In Yapko, M.D. (ed.) **Brief Approaches to Treating Anxiety and Depression**. New York: Brunner/Mazel.

Stern, R. and Marks, I. (1973) Brief and prolonged flooding. **Archives of General Psychiatry** 28, 270–276.

Stuart, R.B. (1969) Operant–interpersonal treatment of marital discord. **Journal of Consulting and Clinical Psychology** 33, 675–682.

Wegner, D.M. (1994) **White Bears and Other Unwanted Thoughts: Suppression, Obsession, and the Psychology of Mental Control**. New York: Guildford Press.

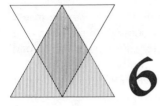 **6**

Handing Over
Generalisation and maintenance of self-management skills

Anni Telford and Andy Farrington

Key issues

- The concept of generalisation
- The importance of generalisation in effective interventions
- Strategies for increasing generalisation
- The importance of self-maintenance
- Strategies for increasing self-management

Introduction

The work clients do between sessions and after seeing the therapist are as important as the work done in session. This chapter, which looks at generalisation and self-maintenance, helps the reader gain an understanding of these two vitally important areas and describes strategies which they can employ to maximise their client's chances of achieving and maintaining change.

Generalisation

Jenny, a 20-year-old student, was referred suffering from a very severe insect phobia. The problem was so bad during the spring and summer months that she was virtually house bound, and had failed her University course because she had missed many of the lectures and had been unable to attend her examinations. Jenny told how, as a young girl, she had watched her mother and aunt panic at the sight of bees and wasps. They would scream and run away whenever these particular insects came near them. Jenny had quickly learned this pattern of behaviour from watching her relatives (vicarious learning; Bandura 1969) and she told how, by the age of 10, she had a bee and wasp phobia.

By the age of 12, Jenny stated that she started to respond in the same way to any insect that buzzed, including flies and bluebottles. By the age of 13 it was any fly or flying insect (except for butterflies, moths and spiders) that invoked her fears regardless of whether it buzzed or not. She then reported how one afternoon she was sitting in the house and noticed what she thought was a beetle on the floor. When she went to kill the beetle it flew away (Jenny was unaware that many beetles can fly), after this incident she noticed her fear occurring whenever she saw an insect (still excluding moths, butterflies and spiders) whether it was flying or not.

She said she was not afraid of butterflies, moths and spiders because they were physically different, one lot had large soft wings and the others spun webs. Jenny's fears had generalised from bees and wasps to flying, buzzing insects to flying insects to crawling insects, but she was still able to discriminate between these sets of insects, and butterflies, spiders and moths.

Whaley and Malott (1971: 175) state that:

> Generally, when two stimuli are physically very similar, considerable generalization will occur between such stimuli and good discrimination behavior will be difficult to establish. If two stimuli are completely different, there may be only a small amount of stimulus generalization between them, and a good discrimination will be established easily.
>
> As may be seen from the preceding account, *generalization is the opposite of discrimination.*

Generalisation occurs when stimuli all share certain properties or similarities; they are then said to belong to a stimulus class. The more dissimilar the stimuli the less likely generalisation is to occur as discrimination between them is easier. In the case of Jenny the stimulus class was any insect which might fly and does not have large soft wings or spin webs. With Jenny it is easy to define the stimulus class that provoked her phobic response and it may seem a simple example, however, complex social situations can become stimulus classes.

Consider Gourmail who came along because she was having problems at work. She had recently been promoted to managerial level and had self-referred because she found she was unable to delegate work and had problems telling staff when they had not performed well. The origin of her problem could be traced to her childhood, when it had been reinforced by her parents that it was not good for little girls to be too assertive in the home. She had experienced problems firstly in her social life whenever she had to be assertive and now this had generalised into the work setting.

Delegation and giving negative feedback had joined the response class of assertive situations.

Just as generalisation can work in widening the number of stimuli that can invoke a fear response, it is important to consider it when attempting to help clients overcome their difficulties. By a careful examination of clients' fears and anxieties, it is possible to identify response classes and most hierarchies, for exposure programmes, are built around a single response class. We can assume that a certain amount of generalisation will occur across the stages of the hierarchy. However, if we incorrectly assume that a stimuli belongs to a response class, when it in fact belongs to another, then no generalisation will occur. An example of this is the case of Mike.

Mike initially presented with a severe social anxiety problem. He was seen by a community psychiatric nurse (CPN) who worked hard giving him anxiety management training. The CPN also used role-playing with Mike for the situation that caused him most anxiety, which was meeting and talking to women in social situations. He dutifully carried out an exposure programme that focused on this aspect of his difficulties. He was discharged when he was able to mix socially with women. Indeed, at the point of discharge he had been seeing a woman friend regularly for 6 weeks. Unfortunately, the CPN had decided that his problems at work were of the same response class as meeting women and thought that generalisation would occur. Mike, however, discovered that this did not happen. After only 3 weeks Mike came back to see the CPN as he was still having problems at work. He had been promoted just prior to seeing the CPN to head of a department in the civil service and was finding it extremely difficult in meetings when he had to present his department's work. The formal work setting was not similar enough in nature to the more relaxed social situation for generalisation to occur and Mike was unable to transfer his new-found confidence into the meetings.

Self-maintenance

A major target of any cognitive behavioural intervention is for the client to become independent of the professional helper, to internalise the strategies and become self-maintaining. This can be viewed as the client's ability to understand the principles behind his/her programme and implement them independently of seeing the helper. It is instrumental in relapse prevention, for if the client fails to self-maintain and returns to old patterns of behaving, then it is probable that the initial problem will re-emerge.

George had come to see a CPN after a serious car crash. He had suffered bad injuries, but after 3 months in hospital had made a full recovery. He told the CPN that he now found himself unable to drive his car or travel as a passenger in the car when his wife was driving it. The CPN, after a thorough assessment, helped George draw up an exposure programme with the following steps:

1. Sit in the CPN's car whilst stationary.
2. Sit in his own car whilst stationary.
3. Travel as a back-seat passenger in the CPN's car on quiet country roads.
4. Travel as a back-seat passenger in the family car on quiet country roads.
5. Travel as a back-seat passenger in the CPN's car on busy roads/on the motorway.
6. Travel as a front-seat passenger in the CPN's car on quiet country roads.
7. Travel as a front-seat passenger in the family car on quiet country roads.
8. Travel as a front-seat passenger in the CPN's car on busy roads/on the motorway.
9. Travel as a front-seat passenger in the family car on busy roads/on the motorway.
10. Drive the family car for short distances on quiet country roads.
11. Drive the family car for long distances on quiet country roads.
12. Drive the family car for short distances on busy roads/on the motorway.
13. Drive the family car for long distances on busy roads/on the motorway.

This 13-step plan was agreed by George and appeared on the surface to be comprehensive. George was also taught relaxation exercises and some cognitive coping strategies for use during his exposure sessions, including the use of positive cue cards and hyperventilation control exercises. His wife agreed to participate and support George during the programme. All went well and George was discharged by the CPN after he had been driving the car on the motorway as part of his homework for a week. He reported that he felt much better and now experienced only very mild anxiety when driving on the motorway and none at all when he was driving on quiet country roads. He was given a follow-up appointment for 2 months time.

At the follow-up, George reluctantly admitted that he was no longer driving the family car and could only travel as a passenger on quiet country roads. The CPN asked how this had happened and George reported that, just after his discharge, the car had required some repairs and had gone into the garage for a week. When the car returned he had experienced an upsurge of anxiety and had avoided driving the car apart from short trips around their village for another week. He had arranged to go to London to visit some relatives the following week and had intended to drive, however, he was so anxious on the morning of the trip that they had arranged to travel by train instead. On their return from London he had managed to persuade his wife to drive on their outings as he wanted 'to have a drink'. When his wife had next suggested a trip which involved the motorway he chose to stay at home and thus, gradually, through lack of self-maintenance, his fears had re-established themselves.

George's case illustrates the dangers of not preparing clients adequately prior to discharge for self-maintenance. Once new patterns of behaviour have been initiated, it is essential that the client continue to practise them until they are firmly established. Once they are established, they are then maintained by their normal consequences. In George's case this might have been the pleasure of being an independent driver able to gain enjoyment from visiting friends and relatives.

Relationships

Kottler (1991: 77) suggests 'Power comes with the territory of being a therapist, whether we like it or not', yet if therapy is to be successful, it must help the client to assume his/her own power, in other words to become his/her own therapist. Thus if the client is to generalise his/her gains and self-maintain, the balance of perceived power must shift from being invested (by the client) in the therapist to being invested in the client him/herself. This is an essential component of the therapeutic relationship, this subtle movement of power from therapist to client. Traditional views of cognitive behaviour therapy have tended to ignore the nature of power within the therapeutic relationship (Lang 1969; Eysenck 1975) viewing the therapist rather like a neutral but supportive educator. Piasecki and Hollan (1987: 141–142) suggest that:

> ... the therapist in cognitive therapy takes on the role of a teacher ... in a similar way to a clinical researcher working with a bright graduate student. ... Our stance is that of an expert, with specific and delimited areas of competence closely related to methodology. ... Traditionally valued therapist characteristics (e.g. warmth, genuineness and empathy) are probably useful, but we see them as being far from sufficient.

However, Fennel and Teasdale (1987) and Simons et al. (1984) suggest that there are some client characteristics that transcend the skills of the therapist and are indicative of enduring and positive outcomes, whilst Jacobson (1989: 89) states that:

> In addition to the healing potential of an interpersonal relationship which is not plagued by discord and disruption, the therapeutic relationship often provides depressed clients with an opportunity to

explore new modes of interpersonal behaviour in a safe inter-personal environment. To the extent that the relationship fails to replicate previous dysfunctional patterns, and when new more adaptive modes of behaving are met with success, the client may be ready for the first time to promote response generalization through venturing forth with these new behaviors into the natural environment.

There are many other workers who support Jacobson's position on the importance of the therapeutic relationship, some of whom are highly influential in this field (Beck et al. 1979; Arnkoff 1983), and it is this position that will be emphasised when examining factors that potentiate generalisation and self-management.

Likeability, similarity, credibility, nurturance and friendliness have all been identified by Shelton and Levy (1981) as important factors affecting the interpersonal influence of the therapist, whilst Schaap et al. (1993: 145), drawing from a variety of workers, suggest that the characteristics that clients see as important and that correlate well with positive outcome are:

- a person with whom I can discuss my personal problems and who helps me understand them,
- emotional warmth and understanding,
- a sympathetic and powerful personality,
- the experience of support and comfort,
- offering advice.

The relationship within cognitive behaviour therapy (CBT) has been described by Beck et al. (1979) as being collaborative in nature, suggesting that therapist and client work together to solve problems and overcome difficulties. Gordon and Marlett (1981) put forward the notion of the relationship being collegial rather than hierarchical in nature, with power shared equally between the client and the therapist. However, these notions of collaboration and collegiality, whilst useful, require further analysis if we are to begin to deal with the nature of power within the therapeutic relationship.

Schaap et al. (1993) identify five main types of power within the therapeutic relationship:

1. Expert power.
2. Referent power.
3. Legitimate power.
4. Informational power.
5. Ecological power.

1. Expert power

Here power is invested in the expert who has, or is perceived by the client to have, the knowledge and skills necessary to resolve problems, which the client has been unable to resolve by themselves.

2. Referent power

When the client experiences dissonance between how they are and how they wish to be, they will try to reduce the discomfort experienced. The difference between myself as I am and myself as I wish to be is based in part on comparisons between self and others. The therapist gains referent power through the level of attractiveness, empathy and social model that they offer the client.

3. Legitimate power

As it suggests, the term 'legitimate power' is to do with societal roles and their various functions. The client, by accepting the power division within therapy, accepts the legitimate power of the therapist and thus accepts his/her suggestions and directions as appropriate.

4. Informational power

The therapist holds knowledge and information, which the client perceives s/he requires to overcome his/her problem.

5. Ecological power

This refers to the therapist's ability to influence the client's environment through encouragement to engage in alternative activities, manipulation of the actual environment or through encouraging relevant others within the client's environment to behave in some way that is different towards the client. The following case example attempts to demonstrate how these notions of collaboration and collegiality can be seen and analysed when working with a client.

Mrs Brown was seen after being referred with a severe needle phobia, which had come to light when she had been diagnosed by her general practitioner as suffering from diabetes. Several attempts had been made at the local hospital to teach Mrs Brown to self-administer both blood sugar tests and insulin by subcutaneous injection, but with no success. As a result the district nurse was visiting the home twice daily to administer Mrs Brown's injections, and both the nurse and Mrs Brown described these visits as both costly in time and extremely traumatic. Mrs Brown was frequently becoming very distressed and tearful whilst the nurse was feeling highly frustrated and angry at her inability to deal with the situation.

Mrs Brown was very anxious and distressed when she arrived at her initial meeting with the therapist, experiencing a panic attack shortly after entering the room, and subsequently becoming very weepy and threatening to leave. When this was gently explored by the therapist, Mrs Brown spoke of her fear of being bullied into giving herself the injections and being forced to stick needles into herself as exposure. She recounted some popular misconceptions about CBT in the form of a 'friend of a friend' who had supposedly been forced by a therapist to sit in a room full of cats on her first visit for a cat phobia. It was important, if Mrs Brown was to overcome her anxiety about treatment and hopefully her problem with needles, to spend time at this point explaining clearly to her the nature of exposure treatment (Marks 1987) and her ultimate control over the process of exposure. The therapist, stating she understood Mrs Brown's fears at being forced into doing something she was afraid of, firstly reassured her that no one would force or push her to do anything she was not prepared to do. She went on to explain that the therapy would go as slowly or as quickly as she, rather than the therapist, wished. Finally she emphasised that the therapist would be there to support her and help her sort out her own treatment programme. Mrs Brown immediately appeared much more relaxed when she felt that she would be in control of the therapy and began to inquire what the therapist knew about diabetes. The therapist admitted honestly that she was fairly ignorant of this medical condition, but also indicated that she was willing to learn about it and about what Mrs Brown would have to do to keep control of her blood sugar levels. The rest of the session was spent with Mrs Brown explaining the condition to the therapist and describing in as much detail as she could what was expected of her. The session ended with mutual homework assignments. Mrs Brown agreed to read a short handout on exposure, its effectiveness and use. The therapist agreed to read a handout on diabetes and its treatment, which the district nurse had given Mrs Brown. The next appointment was arranged and Mrs Brown left feeling much calmer, saying on her way out of the door 'I really think we can crack this stupid needle thing'.

In this example, the therapist demonstrated collaboration and collegiality by her willingness firstly to listen to the client's immediate anxiety rather than rush ahead with an assessment, which, at that point, could only have distressed the client further. Had she done so it could possibly have resulted in Mrs Brown leaving therapy immediately. She would have exercised too much legitimate power at the expense of referent power. She then went on to describe how she could only assist Mrs Brown with her own treatment, thus successfully handing power over to the client, whilst at the same time retaining her expert power and informational power base. She also admitted her ignorance on a topic which the client knew a great deal about, thus assuming the position of student to Mrs Brown's expert and giving Mrs Brown expert power. The client's parting statement was a telling one, which highlighted the nature of collegiality and collaboration within CBT.

Greenberg (1983) suggests that a feeling of active participation within the client is related to therapy outcome. By fostering active participation and client control, the therapist in this example directly involved the client, from the initial session, in the therapy process.

The following case example demonstrates how active participation can be encouraged towards the later stages of therapy and can prepare the way for generalisation and self-maintenance.

Ken, a 56-year-old headmaster, survived a fairly major heart attack. Prior to this he weighed 17 stone, a lot for a man only 5 foot 7 inches in height. He was referred after he had been unable to lose weight on the diet given him by the hospital dietician. During therapy he had managed to lose $3\frac{1}{2}$ stone, but to do this he had avoided many of the social situations where he had previously enjoyed eating and drinking. His therapist, David, was concerned that, although Ken had reached the target weight negotiated between them, on discharge he would return to his previous lifestyle and quickly regain the weight he had lost. The session described here was to have been the penultimate session.

David:	How do you see the past 3 months? Are you pleased with your progress or ...
Ken:	I'm delighted really ... yes delighted. ... I never really thought I'd be able to do it.
David:	Yes, you've done really well ... you should be pleased with yourself.
Ken:	I am pleased ...
David:	We need to start thinking about discharge ... do you think you've reached all the targets you wanted to ... ?
Ken: (hesitantly)	I suppose so. ... I've lost the weight ...
David:	But I sense you sound a little ... well, not worried ... but something's there?
Ken:	I've lost weight before ... 3 years before this heart trouble I lost 2 stone ... but then things went to pot and I put it back on.
David:	And you're concerned that'll happen again?
Ken:	Yes, yes ... all this hard work. ... I don't want to see it go to waste.
David:	So what can we do to try to make sure that doesn't happen?
Ken:	I really don't know. ... I was rather hoping that you'd have some ideas ... perhaps if I saw you every fortnight instead of weekly – a sort of top-up session?
David:	Okay. We can do that for four sessions. What else do you suggest?

(After a short silence)

Ken:	I didn't get on very well with the control exercises you suggested. With me it seems to be all or nothing. ... I can't just have a little bit. I seem to always go overboard.
David:	Do you think going back over the control exercises would help you?
Ken:	I hope so.
David:	Alright, we'll go back over them before you go and spend the first few top-up sessions on them as well. Is there anything else you think we can try?
Ken:	I feel I need to make more of an effort to change the rest of my life. I mean to get exercise but I end up in front of the television. ... I don't know what to do.... I've spent most of my life avoiding exercise.
David:	Perhaps you feel a bit out of your depth where sport and exercise is concerned?
Ken:	That's right. I don't know where to start.
David:	Well, let's start where you feel safest. What sports and activities did you enjoy when you were younger?
Ken:	Swimming ... I liked swimming ... and I used to enjoy walking when my wife was alive, but now I don't seem to have anyone to go walking with. My life centres around the pub and visiting friends for dinner, or going out to dinner with my son and family.
David:	It sounds as though you need someone to share these activities with if you're to enjoy them and keep them up?
Ken: (smiling)	Yes ... I'd feel a bit foolish going walking or swimming on my own ... people might wonder what I was up to! (laughs)
David:	Well, you could join the Ramblers. That way you'd meet people and have someone experienced to go out with. How does that sound?
Ken:	I'll give it a try.... One of the secretaries at the school was a member. She and her husband went out most weekends ... I suppose I could go to the local swimming club ... they have an over-fifties session on a Wednesday morning.
David:	That sounds as though you've already made some enquiries.
Ken:	Well it's been playing on my mind. ... I'm also worried about the drinking. ... How do you turn down a pint? (laughs)
David:	That's something we can look at, what thoughts make it difficult for you to turn down a pint. ... We could develop some coping statements for you to try, and role-play it. Perhaps when you feel more confident at it we could pop down the local and see how you manage?
Ken:	Sounds good to me. ... I've avoided the pub for ages.

As can be seen from the dialogue between Ken and David, the therapist attempts to steer Ken towards making his own decisions about the way he can tackle the problems rather than immediately suggesting what he could do. That is not to say that the therapist would not be directive if required but rather that, wherever possible, he guides the client towards finding his own solutions to the problems and active participation in the therapy process. Thus, the therapeutic relationship can be used as a tool in its own right to encourage clients to generalise and self-maintain.

Strategies

In the introduction it was emphasised that the therapeutic relationship itself is a strong medium for creating therapeutic change. In this section this theme will be continued and developed through the examination of specific therapist actions, which can promote generalisation and self-maintenance. However, it is important to note that, whilst generalisation and self-maintenance are seen as being important aspects of the middle and closing stages of any intervention, if they are to be successfully developed, the therapist must start thinking about them from the very first contact and must monitor their interactions with the client from day one to ensure that generalisation and self-maintenance will be enhanced. It is therefore essential that all stages of therapy are examined in an attempt to promote generalisation and self-maintenance.

Encourage self-direction

This can be started from the first session when the therapist can make space to allow the client to tell his/her own story. Obviously there are set pieces of data that are required if the therapist is to make an assessment and produce a reasonable plan of action, but wherever it is possible, the therapist can allow the client to tell his/her own story. This also helps establish the referent power and trust required for change.

A second strategy for encouraging self-direction is an in-depth examination of the current situation, which highlights the advantages and disadvantages within it, how the client perceives and thinks about the situation and the discomfort they are experiencing. Schaap et al. (1993: 44) suggests that:

> These interventions represent a first attempt against demoralization and should inform the client about his or her own control over the content and the processes of treatment.

The following dialogue, taken from a client who had been referred after a heart attack for lifestyle counselling, gives an example of how this can be done.

Therapist: Can you tell me a little more about how the current situation is affecting your life?

Client: Well, I don't get home until eight or nine most nights and I leave the house around seven every morning.

Therapist: How does that affect your family life?

Client: Mary, my wife, says she never sees me. I know I should spend more time with the kids. ... It's difficult setting priorities ... work pulls one way and the family pulls the other.

Therapist: So it's fair to say that, if things carry on as they are, your relationships with your wife and family will suffer. Let's put this down here under negative effects.

Client: But if I didn't work so hard, the money would stop.

Therapist: Right. Well, we can put that down under positive effects here.

Client: The other problem is my weight and health. There's pressure to have business lunches with clients but I just don't have time to exercise.

Therapist: What exercise do you want to do?

Client: I used to be a keen footballer and I played badminton for the county as a youngster. ... That's all gone now.

Therapist: Shall we put that in the negative column?

Client: Yes. ... I really miss my football.

(The therapist and client continue working until there are several entries in the positive column and a considerable number in the negative column. The therapist and client then go on to identify priorities for change and elicit cognitions about those priorities.)

Therapist: I think I have a clearer idea now of how things are in your life.

Client: Yes. ... It's been useful, but I'd no idea things were so bad. No wonder I had the heart attack. ... This looks terrible.

Therapist: I don't know about terrible, I think that's a good example of magnification, but it gives us a clear picture of how things are. Perhaps now we need to look at how you want things to be and move forward from this point.

Client: I don't know where to start.

Therapist: Well, a lot of this seems to me to be tied up with the amount of time you spend at work ... and perhaps the way you think about work?

Client: Okay ... yes it does. Perhaps if we started looking at how I can change how I think about work and the amount of time I spend there ... as a priority really. ... If I don't change those, then nothing will get done.

Therapist: So let's spend a little time looking at that. What sort of things do you say to yourself about work?

Client: (after a thoughtful silence) I think the main idea that I have is that I've got to get everything right ... absolutely perfect ... otherwise. ...

Therapist: Otherwise?

Client: Otherwise ... I'll be no good. I keep going over stuff ... again and again ... to make sure it's right. That includes all the stuff my staff produce.

It's a big office, over twelve staff, and all this checking to make sure it's right before it goes off to head office . . . it all takes time.

Therapist: So I think we may have to work on some cognitive and behavioural strategies to help you examine this and make work less time consuming. . . . I think we need to look at what you think will happen if you make a mistake.

Setting goals

Many clients come into therapy after several failed attempts to overcome their problems and take control of their lives. Their perception of self and ability to cope may therefore be at a fairly low ebb. If we as therapists wish clients to take control of their therapy in an effort to encourage generalisation and self-maintenance, it seems essential that we increase their perceptions of coping and self-efficacy. Setting unrealistic goals for a client who is already demoralised and demobilised can only further add to the burden of the problems they face. Failure when attempting home-work assignments further reinforces in the client their inability to overcome their problems without the support of the therapist. If goals are to assist the client in breaking the failure barrier, they must be realistic and achievable.

This may require setting a series of sub-goals for clients who are seriously demoralised and working with them on the cognitive set that prevents them from succeeding at homework tasks. For example, if the client is thinking something along the lines of 'What's the point, I'm never going to get over this', it is pertinent to address this negative prediction of the future before s/he leaves to attempt the homework task.

Consider the following case report. Mrs Simms had been complaining of severe lowering of mood and, by the time she was seen by the counsellor in her local doctor's general practice, she was doing very little. She did not get out of bed most days until two or three in the afternoon and then spent most of the day sitting in front of the television. She was not washing or dressing herself, the house was seriously neglected and she had not been outside for over 4 weeks. She had lost 3 stones in weight and was living on a diet of convenience foods, which her nextdoor neighbour was providing for her. The counsellor was very concerned about Mrs Simms poor physical and psychological health, and felt that some serious action needed to be taken if an admission to the local psychiatric hospital was to be avoided. She spent one and a half hours working with Mrs Simms and then set her the following homework:

1. Get up at nine o'clock each day.
2. Have a shower or bath.
3. Get dressed.
4. Collect your automatic negative thoughts in the diary sheet provided.
5. Go for a walk of 15 minutes duration.

6. Eat at least two proper meals each day.

The counsellor was surprised when Mrs Simms did not turn up for her session the following week and brought the problem to supervision, where it was suggested that she had set unrealistic and unachievable goals for a client who was severely depressed, thus compounding the failure of Mrs Simms to get to grips with her problems yet again. The counsellor arranged to visit Mrs Simms in her home and at that meeting discussed with her the feelings of hopelessness which Mrs Simms had experienced when the homework was set. The following dialogue addressed Mrs Simm's thoughts at the time.

Mrs Simms: I just thought here's another one who doesn't understand. . . . I'll never be able to do all of that and I'll never get over this. What's the point in struggling on?

Counsellor: Well, one thing's right there. I didn't fully understand how you were at the time. If I had I might have asked you what you thought you could manage ... and I could have helped you work on any thoughts you had which might be instrumental in not achieving the negotiated goals. But I think there's a problem with the last thing you said, 'I'll never get over this'. You seem to be turning my mistake into a kind of all-round failure on your part, you're personalising and magnifying something which is my mistake.

(Mrs Simms looks thoughtful for a few minutes.)

Mrs Simms: I see what you mean. . . .

Counsellor: So we need to look at what you think you can do and work on those self-defeating cognitions before we set any more homework.

The following homework was then agreed:

1. Get up at one o'clock rather than two.
2. Collect automatic negative thoughts that focus on the hopelessness of the situation.
3. Read one page of a romantic novel each day (an activity Mrs Simms had previously enjoyed).

The counsellor then spent time working with Mrs Simms on cognitions, which might stop her achieving her goals.

Mrs Simms was able to carry out all of her homework assignments and went on to make good progress.

By setting realistic and achievable goals in the second session and working on Mrs Simms self-defeating cognitions, the counsellor was able to recover her position and help Mrs Simms see that she could effect change in her life. She was also able to use this as an example of how Mrs Simms herself could break down problems in to smaller chunks and sub-goals in preparation for discharge later on.

Reinforcement of self-help and self-reinforcement skills

As was stated at the beginning of this chapter, the aim of the therapist, if they wish their clients to self-maintain, is to assist their clients to take control of the therapy. Part of this process can be achieved by the constant encouragement of self-help skills and client problem solving.

One method of reinforcing self-help skills, particularly with clients who require some form of exposure treatment, is the use of self-exposure programmes. This, Marks (1987) suggests, can be particularly useful with clients who have phobic or obsessive compulsive problems. With clients experiencing obsessive compulsive problems, self-imposed response prevention can also be employed. Marks suggests that 'imposing external constraints achieves little in the long run' (p. 493). It is important, however, when the client has successfully undertaken such an exercise, to ensure that they are reinforced for his/her hard work and effort in undertaking the homework. Many clients are unable to see their achievements, as they believe they should be able to perform the tasks in the first instance, that no special effort is involved on their part when facing up to situations that provoke a phobic response. Their negative cognitive schema prevents them from self-reinforcing. The following dialogue emphasises how the therapist can reinforce a client's achievement when she is belittling her own efforts at performing a particularly fearful homework assignment.

Therapist: How did the homework go?
Client: Once I plucked up the courage to get on with this it was really alright. I managed everything I set myself.
Therapist: That's excellent.... You've done really well with this. Last week when we spoke, you said this was going to be really difficult and you were very worried about it.
Client: But it's nothing really.... Everyone apart from me could have managed it. It's stupid that I couldn't do it in the first place.
Therapist: Let's look at what's going on here with your thinking. Last week you were really frightened about exposing yourself to this and we had to spend time working on some strategies to help you get started with it. ... Now today you're saying it was nothing really? I don't quite understand this. How difficult was it last week?
Client: You know it was really difficult.
Therapist: So why is it suddenly nothing?
Client: Well it's not nothing.... I did do it and I was really scared.
Therapist: Good. You did really do it ... all by yourself ... there was no one there at the time to help you through it.
Client: Yes, I know ... but anyone could do it.
Therapist: I know some clients who couldn't have done it ... some clients who would have needed my support first time in that situation.

Client: Yes?

Therapist: Yes. There are some clients who couldn't manage what you did.

Client: Yes, but they're clients.... Any normal person could have done it.

Therapist: But your fear was real and you faced it. Let's put this into a different context.... In your job, you have to deal with all kinds of dogs ... is that right?

Client: Yes.

Therapist: So you deal with big dogs ... German Shepherds and Rottweilers and such like?

Client: Yes ... but I'm not scared of dogs.

Therapist: That's right. You're not scared of dogs.... You've frequently said to me that it's not the dog, it's the way you think about them and treat them that makes a dog misbehave. So you think dogs are nothing to be frightened of ... but I know quite a few so-called normal people that would be really scared to handle big dogs the way you do.

Client: So?

Therapist: If one of those people who were frightened of dogs came along and plucked up the courage to do what you do with them, what would you think of them?

Client: I'd think they were really brave.

Therapist: Even though you and I know that dogs are not in themselves dangerous?

Client: Yes.

Therapist: But you were really frightened about what you set yourself as homework, even though I knew it wasn't really dangerous to do.

Client: (after a short silence) So what you're saying is that it doesn't matter if it's dangerous or not, if you are frightened of something and pluck up the courage to do it, then that's an achievement?

Therapist: That's what I'm saying. You've got one rule for yourself and one for other people here.

Client: Yes, I see that now.

Therapist: So let's start again.... How was the homework?

Client: It was really difficult, but I managed to do it and I'm rather proud of myself.

Therapist: You need to watch that tendency to put yourself and your achievements down. When we finish therapy you'll need to be able to pick yourself up on these negative ideas, and praise yourself when you achieve something.

In this instance, the therapist uses the opportunity to demonstrate to the client that she had achieved something, which, for her, was very difficult but she then went on through her automatic negative thoughts to negate her own achievement. The therapist continues and uses the example to prepare the client for self-maintenance once they have been discharged.

External relationship use

The therapeutic relationship is an intense one, with the therapist holding a highly influential position in the client's life. The therapist, by his/her use of ecological power, can encourage others in the client's life firstly to assist the client in overcoming his/her problems and secondly to help the client self-maintain. This use of external relationships may go some way to reduce the importance of the therapist and eventually the loss involved in the therapist's withdrawal at discharge. There are a variety of ways that this can be achieved including:

- Using family and relevant others as co-therapists.
- Using relevant others as agents of reinforcement.
- Encouraging relevant others to change their own behaviours to reduce the likelihood of relapse.

The following case examples go some way to demonstrating how this can be achieved, however in each case an assessment of the ability and willingness of relevant others to become involved is essential.

Using relevant others as co-therapists

With only limited training in exposure principles, relevant others can be encouraged to act as co-therapists in exposure programmes for those clients who are unable, initially, to self-expose.

Barlow et al. (1984) suggests that agoraphobia improved more in clients who had involved their spouses as exposure co-therapists than those who had not, and this supports the work of Mathews et al. (1981). The effectiveness of unrelated partners was demonstrated by Ross (1980) who used former successfully treated phobics as co-therapists. If the client is unlikely to have contact with the co-therapist after discharge, then there may be little benefit in terms of self-maintenance. It is fairly easy to see how one might recruit a spouse to fulfil the role but a variety of relevant others can be employed as the following example shows.

Sally was a bright and articulate 20-year-old who was referred with problems controlling her eating. She tended to binge on chocolate, cakes, biscuits and other carbohydrate-rich foods. A self-control programme was initiated and this involved an element of exposure to the binge foods. Sally was able to expose to the binge foods in the clinic with the therapist present and was also able to achieve self-exposure in the clinic without the therapist present. When asked to carry out self-exposure in the home, however, Sally reported that in the first week she had binged on the exposure foods three times and was too fearful thereafter to continue the self-exposure programme at home. Having achieved self-exposure in the clinic, the therapist decided that it might be a retrograde step to then start with therapist-controlled exposure in the home and an alternative solution was sought. This came in the shape of one of Sally's friends who had been supportive to Sally in the past. The friend attended two training sessions with the therapist who taught her how to:

1. Withhold reassurance about her weight from Sally.
2. How to prompt coping statements.
3. How to simply challenge automatic negative thoughts.
4. How to prompt self-reinforcing statements.

Exposure was recommenced at home, first with her friend in the same room, then with her friend in the next room. The next step involved her friend arriving some time into the session, then phoning during the session and, finally, Sally phoning her friend once the exposure was successfully completed.

The therapist utilised this friend further when preparing for discharge and encouraged her to help Sally in situations post-discharge in which Sally felt she was most likely to binge.

Using relevant others as agents of reinforcement

Matt was a 7-year-old boy referred with temper tantrums. He was disruptive at home, at school, with his grandparents and at cubs whenever he did not get his own way. The social worker found it fairly easy to teach Matt's mother techniques to reward Matt when he was behaving well and ways of dealing with him when he was having a tantrum. She also worked with Matt's mother on challenging her feelings of guilt and failing Matt as a mother. The problem subsided at home and Matt was discharged, however, after only 2 weeks, the social worker was again contacted by Matt's mother who reported that Matt was behaving reasonably well at home but the main problem was reoccurring outside of the home. This had started when Matt visited his maternal grandparents and stopped over without his parents. He had thrown a temper tantrum when he was not allowed to stay up to watch television. His grandparents had responded by allowing him to stay up. He then threw a tantrum the next day at school which had resulted in the teacher reading him a story. The next evening he had thrown a tantrum at cubs and Matt's mother was asked to come and collect him as the cub leader was unable to deal with him.

The social worker correctly deduced that generalisation had not occurred beyond Matt's immediate family and home environment. S/he asked Matt's mother to contact the school and the cub leader to see if they would be willing to help Matt with his problem. Matt's grandparents were also contacted and asked for assistance. All agreed to attend a training session at Matt's home. The social worker taught the group the same techniques for reinforcing positive behaviour and ignoring tantrums, which had been so successful for Matt's mother, and worked with everyone on the types of cognitive distortions that might prevent them from carrying out the programme. They agreed to implement the strategies over the following 2 weeks and then meet back at Matt's home. All reported that Matt had attempted to throw temper tantrums with them but that order was quickly restored when the techniques were implemented. Matt was then discharged and at 6-month follow-up, Matt himself reported that he had not had a tantrum and that he was much happier.

This example, using a child, is easy to see, but it is also possible to use relevant others as reinforcement agents with adults.

Madeline was a 44-year-old woman who had problems controlling her diet. This was particularly relevant as Madeline was an insulin-dependent diabetic. The district nurse who visited Madeline noted that Madeline's main pleasure came from food, and that her husband and adult son, who lived at home, paid little attention to her, apart from nagging her when she overindulged in sweets and cakes. She taught Madeline some self-control skills, which were reasonably successful at first, however, Madeline then began to slip back into her old eating patterns. At this point, the district nurse taught both husband and son some simple reinforcement techniques, to spend more time talking to Madeline when she wasn't eating, to visit the cinema with her, and accompany her to visits to her daughter and children who lived some way away. They were also to praise Madeline's control when she managed to resist sweets and cakes, but were to reduce eye contact and conversation with her when she succumbed. After 3 weeks, Madeline reported a dramatic decrease in her consumption of sweets. This improvement maintained up to discharge.

Encouraging relevant others to change their own behaviours to reduce the likelihood of relapse

Marks (1987) reports many incidents where family behaviours have been in collusion with the rituals of clients with obsessive compulsive problems, undertaking excessive washing or checking, for example, and this can be seen in many other problem areas. If the client is to self-maintain, then the therapist must take into consideration the behaviour of others as variables that are likely to encourage relapse and use their environmental power to influence those behaviours.

Jim was a 62-year-old man who had retired after a stroke left him partially paralysed down the left side. He was referred to a community psychiatric nurse for help some 2 years later after he had repeatedly presented at his doctor's surgery complaining of various aches and pains for which the doctor could find no physical cause. On assessment, Jim appeared anxious and rather low in mood. He was unclear why he had been referred to a CPN when he believed he was suffering from some physical illness that his doctor would not tell him about or indeed could not diagnose. He repeated a long list of physical symptoms to the CPN, all of which appeared to be the physical manifestations of anxiety, which Jim was misinterpreting as evidence of his imminent demise, either from a heart attack or another stroke. After an assessment, the CPN instigated some anxiety-management training, paying particular attention to the physical symptomatology of anxiety and the way Jim was misinterpreting them.

Jim, in session, appeared to understand and accept the training the CPN gave. However, he found it difficult to retain any of the concepts in a meaningful way between sessions, and returned each week to report that things were not improving and that he felt as bad as ever. The CPN decided to investigate why Jim was not able to maintain his gains at home by carrying out a home assessment. This revealed that his wife Dorothy had been devastated by Jim's stroke and was now overconcerned about his well-being. She did virtually everything for him in the mistaken belief that he had to take things easy and was constantly checking up on how he felt, and inquiring after his various symptoms. The CPN started to work with Dorothy's anxieties. She had always stayed in the home and had few friends outside of it. Her family had moved away to take up various jobs and Jim was her mainstay in life. She was very worried about what would become of her if Jim suffered another stroke, and became disabled or died. Working gently and in a supportive way, the CPN was able to help Dorothy to explore her automatic negative thoughts and challenge them. These included:

- 'If he dies, I'll never cope on my own'.
- 'If he dies, it will be my fault for not looking after him'.
- 'People who are ill must never exert themselves'.

Eventually Dorothy was able to see how her cognitions led to her over-protection of Jim, and how this was, in fact, more likely to lead to another stroke, as lack of activity had increased both his weight and his blood pressure. The CPN taught Dorothy to avoid asking Jim how he was and rather to encourage him to focus outside his physical symptomatology. Once Dorothy was able to do this, the CPN restarted work with Jim. He was able to maintain his gains between sessions and was discharged some 3 months later. At 6-month follow-up, Dorothy's changed behaviour had allowed Jim to make further improvements and they were planning a cruise to the Canary Islands to celebrate a forthcoming wedding anniversary.

Prepare the client for discharge

In preparing the client for discharge, it is important that the therapist works through with the client what high-risk situations they are likely to come across in their day-to-day environment and help them prepare for:

- Anticipating and facing difficult situations.
- Coping with temporary setbacks.

Preparing for and facing difficult situations

There are four main steps to consider here:

- Identifying new skills and ways of thinking.
- Identifying high-risk situations.

- Developing a plan of action.
- Coping in the situation.

In helping the client identify high-risk situations, the therapist needs to have a sound understanding of the stimuli which trigger the problem. Consider the following case.

Mrs Linda Peters, a 26-year-old married housewife with one child, had been seeing the community psychiatric nurse for help with her anxiety problems, which tended to occur in certain social situations. The conversation here took place during the final session before discharge.

CPN:	We spoke last week of your discharge and how ready you felt for that, how do you feel about it this week?
Mrs Peters:	I still feel fairly confident. ... A bit worried about Christmas, I suppose, if I'm honest about it.
CPN:	I think all clients who are coming up to discharge feel a bit anxious about it.... What particularly is worrying you?
Mrs Peters:	How I'll cope on my own really ... without your support.
CPN:	Let's look at how things have changed for you, and then have a look at Christmas and other situations which you think might be hard to face. But we'll start with the change....
Mrs Peters:	Things have changed, you've shown me how to think about things in a different way.
CPN:	Okay ... so you have new ways of looking at and thinking about things.
Mrs Peters:	Yes ... and I don't avoid doing things any more. You've shown me that facing up to what's scary is better in the long run than trying to wriggle out of things.
CPN:	Anything else?
Mrs Peters:	Relaxation skills.... They were useful ... and the breathing exercises to stop panic developing.
CPN:	Anything else?
Mrs Peters:	I feel better about myself.... I'm as good as anyone else.... You've helped me with that as well ... and the assertion exercises helped. I feel so much better when things get a bit sticky.
CPN:	So there really is quite a difference in things – relaxation skills, thinking differently, not avoiding things, more assertive and feeling better about yourself. ... That's quite a change in ten weeks. ... Quite a lot of new strategies to help you cope with life.
Mrs Peters:	When you add it all up like that ... yes ... it is a big change.
CPN:	Well, perhaps it might help you to cope over the next few weeks if you can recall easily how things have changed. That might stop you slipping back into the problem patterns that brought you here in the first place.
Mrs Peters:	I could make a list and stick it up on the kitchen wall.

CPN:	Excellent. That sounds just the kind of thing I think would be useful. Let's have a think now about what situations might be difficult. You mentioned Christmas?
Mrs Peters:	Yes ... I'm supposed to be having the family over ... all of them ... for Christmas dinner. In the past I've been in an absolute panic about it ... will the food be alright ... what to do with David's mother ... she's so picky about everything. Last year I was completely exhausted by two o'clock and spent all of Boxing Day in bed recovering. It ruins my Christmas every year.
CPN:	Right. It sounds as though you've had a bad time in the past. What can you do this year that would be different? I'll write your ideas down as we discuss it.
Mrs Peters:	I could plan a simpler menu. I was up until 2 a.m. on Christmas morning sorting out bits and pieces, and then spent most of the day cooking.
CPN:	Good idea. What about planning a meal that you could prepare a few days or even weeks before and then freeze?
Mrs Peters:	I could do that with the starters and pudding, but David likes his traditional turkey. I could do the vegetables the day before though.
CPN:	Okay. That sounds like a good compromise. What else could you do?

(Mrs Peters and the CPN then go on to sort out a series of strategies that will help her cope with Christmas, including preparing a cue card beforehand for when things might go wrong, practising her breathing exercises, making time for herself during the day and delegating some of the Christmas tasks to her husband and sister-in-law who will also be coming. Once this is completed, the CPN moves back to try to help her identify other potentially stressful situations.)

CPN:	We've spent a considerable time sorting out Christmas, but can you identify any other danger spots?
Mrs Peters:	(hesitating) There's the staff Christmas party at David's work. That's always an ordeal.
CPN:	Anything else?
Mrs Peters:	We were supposed to go out for dinner with some friends.
CPN:	Anything else?
Mrs Peters:	I always hate the parent–teachers open nights at the school.
CPN:	Anything else?
Mrs Peters:	David's father's birthday.

(They continue to develop a list of situations which Mrs Peters feels will be difficult.)

CPN:	Well, we've got a list of eight potentially difficult situations here. What have you learned from the Christmas example which might be useful?

Mrs Peters: I think the planning aspect.... If you know in advance things might be a bit tricky, you can work out strategies which can help you work your way through.

CPN: Good! You can sit down before you go into a situation and sort it out in your head before you have to meet it. It gives you time to reflect on what new strategies you have and how you can apply them to the situation.

Mrs Peters: But what happens if I have a panic attack? I had one at the office party last year and David was furious because he had to take me home.

CPN: Good question. What have you learned to do about panic attacks?

Mrs Peters: Control my breathing ...

CPN: Right ... and ...

Mrs Peters: Relax into it ... sort out my thinking about what's happening to me and wait for it to pass. That's easy to say here and I have managed to do it during exposure sessions, but my mind goes blank in the real situation.

CPN: Well, maybe cue cards can help here again. You could draw up some small cue cards to carry with you into these situations to remind you what to do if you think you're about to panic.

Mrs Peters: That sounds like a good idea. Yes, I think that would help.

In this example, the CPN has helped the client to identify:

- New skills developed during the therapy sessions.
- Situations that may prove difficult after discharge.
- Strategies to help the client prepare for the situations before entering them.
- Strategies for dealing with panic when in the situations.
- A strategy to remind the client to use her new skills when she feels she is being overwhelmed.

Coping with temporary setbacks

Cognitive techniques can be usefully employed to help clients cope post-discharge and it is suggested that at least one session is devoted primarily to this prior to the discharge point. Many clients, when they experience a temporary setback, find it difficult to deal rationally with the situation, believing that any setback, no matter how small, is a sign of total failure. This belief may result in demoralisation and relapse. By preparing clients for setbacks, it is possible to arm them against this and help clients to see setbacks in proportion. There are two main steps involved in the process: preparation for setbacks, and coping when they occur.

Preparation for setbacks. By telling our clients to expect setbacks to occur, we are strengthening their perception of coping by increasing their understanding of the therapy process. Regardless of how effective cognitive behaviour therapy is, most clients will experience temporary setbacks, at some point after discharge. By explaining this to our clients, we can increase their self-efficacy and thus their potential to deal with the situation. It is far better that the client experiences a constructive thought along the lines of 'I know what's happening. This is what the therapist warned me about' than the more destructive 'It's coming back, just like before'. By explaining that setbacks will probably occur, we can forearm our clients for when the setbacks happen.

Coping with setbacks. It is very easy for clients to fall back into habitual ways of behaving and thinking when setbacks occur. By teaching clients to use cognitive techniques to challenge their negative thinking during setback episodes, we may be able to influence the severity and duration of the period of relapse. The following case example demonstrates how this can be done.

Debbie is a 26-year-old woman who was seen with severe obsessional problems, and the session is just before discharge. The therapist has carefully explained to Debbie that she must expect periods when things do not go to plan and she experiences a re-emergence of her obsessional symptoms.

Therapist: You seem upset by what I've said Debbie?

Debbie: Yes ... yes. ... You seem to be suggesting that it's going to come back ... that's a bit frightening really.

Therapist: Well, I don't think I'm saying that it's going to come back ... but I am saying that you've done very well in therapy and that I want to make sure that you carry on doing well. That means facing up to the idea that there may be hiccups, and times when it may be a case of two steps forward and one back. What we need to do, to make sure you carry on progressing, is prepare for those times. Then, if they do occur, you will not be thrown by them. ... You'll be able to cope with them.

Debbie: I think I understand.

Therapist: Good. ... Let's look at what might go wrong then. ... You mentioned holidays as being very difficult times in the past for you ... when it seemed as though you could get no rest from your thoughts. ... Perhaps we could use that as an example.

Debbie: Yes, I've always had problems with my ruminations on holidays.

Therapist: Right, what sort of thoughts did you have in the past about holidays?

Debbie: Well ... that things are going wrong at home ... the house has caught fire ... or my mum's died and they can't contact me ... (laughs). ... My usual stuff really, but so strong and so persistent.

Therapist: And have you a holiday planned for this coming year?

Debbie: We had planned to go to southern Italy.

Therapist: Okay. ... I want you to close your eyes and imagine that time has rolled by and things are going well ... that you've had no problems and now you're on holiday.

Debbie: (closing her eyes and leaning back in the chair) Right.

Therapist: Describe to me where you are Debbie.

Debbie: On the beach. . . . I'm just lying in the sun . . . relaxing.

Therapist: Right. . . . Now the thought comes into your head that a dreadful accident has happened at home. Your mother is involved, and she's seriously ill in hospital. How do you feel?

Debbie: Okay. . . . I feel okay. . . . You've taught me how to deal with those thoughts.

Therapist: But this one won't go away. . . . It keeps coming back . . . buzzing around your head. . . . Mum's in hospital. Over and over. How do you feel?

Debbie: I can't get rid of the thought?

Therapist: No, it just keeps coming back . . . over and over. (Client starts to look concerned.)

Debbie: I don't like this. . . . I'm starting to become tense.

Therapist: What are you thinking at this point Debbie?

Debbie: How can I control this.

Therapist: Good . . . that's good. . . . You try all the strategies we've gone through: you try thought stopping, you try distraction, you try challenging the idea. Nothing works at first and it takes a good hour or two before you can get things straight. What are you feeling and thinking now?

Debbie: I'm starting to feel really worried now. . . . The thoughts are not very good. . . . I'm in trouble. . . . This hasn't happened before . . . I'll be back to square one. . . . This is just how I was when we started therapy. . . . It hasn't worked.

Therapist: Okay, Debbie, open your eyes. Let's try to work on those last thoughts you were having.

The therapist and Debbie then work together writing down and challenging the thoughts Debbie produced in the imaginal situation. They then produce a diary sheet (Table 6.1).

As can be seen from this example, the therapist uses the same techniques of cognitive restructuring that may have been used at any point in the therapy itself to work through the cognitive component of the setback.

By firstly preparing out clients to expect setbacks and secondly giving them the tools to deal with the setbacks, we can hope to potentiate self-maintenance.

When things do not go as planned

With generalisation the therapist may only realise things have gone wrong when the clients fail to make satisfactory progress. For example, when they are unable to move from one step of an exposure hierarchy to the next and when clients fail to make progress across stimulus classes.

Table 6.1
Rational Challenges Diary

Situation	Thoughts	Challenges	Rational thoughts
Sunbathing and start to ruminate about accidents at home.	I'm in trouble.	What evidence do I have? What would my therapist say?	I was warned about situations like this. It's just a temporary setback.
As above	This hasn't happened before.	Am I exaggerating the importance of events? What is the effect of thinking this way?	Just because it hasn't happened before doesn't make it so desperate. I'm frightening myself thinking like this.
As above	I'm back to square one.	What evidence do I have? Am I condemning myself on a single event?	I have no evidence I'm back to square one. I have loads of new ways of coping with this that I never had before. Just because I've had a setback doesn't mean I'm a failure, it just means I'm the same as everyone else. We all have setbacks.
As above	This is how I was before therapy.	Am I concentrating on my weaknesses and forgetting my strengths?	Yes, I'm not the same as before therapy. I can now use a whole range of strategies to sort this out.
As above	It hasn't worked.	What evidence do I have for this? Am I only paying attention to the bad side of things?	I have lots of evidence that therapy did work. I've worked hard and it's paid off. I've been getting better and better. This morning was excellent, I didn't think of home once.

Failure of self-maintenance on the other hand may only be observed when clients are seen again at follow-up and have slipped back into habitual ways of behaving and thinking.

With clients who have failed to generalise, a careful reassessment of both the clients and the interventions made are required to attempt to ameliorate the situation. This should include a review of the stimulus classes used in any exposure programme, with particular attention paid to their similarities and differences. It is also important to examine variables that may exist within the exposure programme, which are preventing generalisation. For example, has the hierarchy only included accompanied exposure and suddenly moved to self-exposure carried out alone. It is also important to examine the clients' cognitive schemata. Have they slipped into old ways of thinking which have caused the relapse, or have they developed some new set of self-defeating cognitions about the value of continuing with self-maintenance strategies?

In attempting to work out what has happened in failures of self-maintenance, a wider set of variables may need to be addressed. These might include:

- The nature of the power relationship between client and therapist.
- The influence of relevant others on self-maintenance.
- Preparation for self-maintenance (both cognitive and behavioural).
- Reinforcement for changed behaviours (both cognitive and behavioural).
- Reinforcement for habitual behaviours (both cognitive and behavioural).

Consider the following case example.

Gill was an 18-year-old girl who presented with an eating problem. On entry to therapy, she weighed only 6 stone 4 pounds and was 5 feet 8 inches in height. She successfully completed therapy and was discharged after 18 sessions weighing a more appropriate 9 stone 1 pound. She was eating around 2000 calories a day and had successfully altered her faulty cognitions about weight, appearance and worth. At one month follow-up, Gill had maintained well, and was planning to move back out of her parents' home and go back to college, where she had been studying dance and drama prior to her seeking help. Gill cancelled her 3-month follow-up appointment but reported by phone that everything was going well. At 6-month follow-up Gill did attend, she weighed only 6 stones 6 pounds and reported that she was eating around 300 calories a day.

Through careful interviewing and reliance on supervision, the therapist working with the case identified the following factors involved in Gill's relapse:

1. Whilst at home with her parents, her mother had taken responsibility for preparing small but appetising meals for Gill. This was no longer

the case when Gill had to take responsibility for her own catering on return to her shared flat.

2. The students with whom Gill shared a flat were also dance and drama students and the emphasis within the flat was centred on slimness and appearance. They had encouraged Gill to resume dieting on her return to the flat.

3. The practice studio where the dance classes were held were mirror lined and Gill was exposed to seeing her own body in a tight Lycra leotard for at least 2 hours each day. She found she was almost unable to tolerate the images and had started dieting straight after her first dance class.

4. During therapy, Gill had encouraged the therapist to be directive, taking up a fairly helpless position. The male therapist had responded to this in a paternalistic way and had, to a certain extent, encouraged Gill's dependence on him.

5. Whilst Gill had been prepared for discharge, the therapist had prepared her for return to the fairly safe environment within the family home and not to the college environment with its emphasis on appearance and slimness.

As can be seen from this example, both lack of generalisation (items 1 and 5), faulty therapeutic relationship style (item 4), and other variables (items 2 and 3) all worked together to prevent Gill from self-maintaining. She had gone back to her habitual ways of thinking and behaving.

Supervision

The traditional model of supervision within cognitive behavioural therapy tends to focus on the therapist's abilities to:

- Make a detailed assessment.
- Formulate a treatment programme.
- Carry out the treatment programme in a skilled fashion.

It takes little account of therapist variables, the therapeutic relationship and process variables within therapy. This narrow focus approach is insufficient when attempting to address the various factors that can influence the generalisation and self-maintenance of clients. A supervision model, which addresses the process as well as the product of therapy, needs to be sought. Hawkins and Shohet (1993) present a double-matrix model, which can be adapted for use within the cognitive behavioural model. It addresses both the therapy matrix and the supervision matrix, and accounts for both process and product variables.

Within the therapy matrix the model addresses:

(a) The content of the therapy session. This focuses on the client, their attitudes, feelings and beliefs as expressed during the session.
(b) The strategies and interventions used. This focuses on the therapist, their choice of strategies and the skill with which they were applied.
(c) The therapy process and relationships. This focuses on the power variables within the relationship and the therapist's insight into them.

Within the supervisory matrix the model focuses on:

(d) The trainees' reactions to the client. This focuses on the therapist's insight into any attitudes and prejudices that may affect the therapeutic processes.
(e) The supervisory relationship. This focuses on patterns of behaviour within the supervisor–supervisee relationship, which may affect the process of therapy and the development of the therapist.
(f) The supervisor. This focuses on the supervisor's own thoughts and feelings in the here and now and how they reflect on the therapy and the development of the supervisee.

The double matrix of Hawkins and Shohet (1993) allows the examination of all variables within the therapeutic process. It appears to be the most likely vehicle to assist therapists and their supervisors to take on board a full analysis of both therapeutic product and processes.

Ideas for discussion

Whilst accepting the importance of assessing all external variables to control generalisation and self-maintenance, this chapter fails to address issues of gender and ethnic origin within the therapeutic endeavour, as there is little space to address such complex issues within a chapter of this nature. The practitioner is well advised to consider ethnic origin and gender when pondering on generalisation and self-maintenance, as these can be affected by enculturation and family structures. Several texts are therefore suggested in further reading, which would address these issues.

The chapter started with a discussion of the nature of the therapeutic relationship within cognitive behaviour therapy and it is fitting that it should end there. Cognitive behaviourists must wake up to the fact that the notion of the therapist as a neutral onlooker is no longer acceptable within therapy and develop their research strategy to include process as well as product research.

References

Arnkoff, D.B. (1983) Common and specific factors in cognitive therapy. In Lambert, M.J. (ed.) **Psychotherapy and Patient Relationships**. Chicago: Dorsey, pp. 85–125.

Bandura, A. (1969) **Principles of Behavior Modification**. New York: Holt, Rinehart and Winston, Inc.

Barlow, D.H., O'Brien, G.T. and Last, C.G. (1984) Couples treatment of agoraphobia. **Behavior Therapy** 15, 41–58.

Beck, A.T., Rush, A.J., Shaw, B.F. and Emery, G. (1979) **Cognitive Therapy of Depression**. New York: Guilford.

Eysenck, H.J. (1975) Some comments on the relation between A-B status of behaviour therapists and success of treatment. **Journal of Consulting and Clinical Psychology** 43, 86–87.

Fennel, M.J.V. and Teasdale, J.D. (1987) Cognitive therapy for depression: individual differences and the process of change. **Cognitive Therapy and Research** 11, 253–271.

Gordon, J.R. and Marlett, G.A. (1981) Addictive behaviors. In Shelton, J.L. and Levy, R.L. (eds) **Behavioral Assignments and Treatment Compliance: A Handbook of Clinical Strategies**. Champaign, IL: Research, pp. 167–186.

Greenberg, L.S. (1983) Psychotherapy process research. In Walker, C.E. (ed.) **Handbook of Clinical Psychology**. Homewood, IL: Dow Jones–Irwin, pp. 169–204.

Hawkins, P. and Shohet, R. (1993) **Supervision in the Helping Professions**. Milton Keynes: Open University Press.

Jacobson, N.S. (1989) The therapist–client relationship in cognitive behavior therapy: Implications for treating depression. **Journal of Cognitive Psychotherapy: An International Quarterly** 3, 85–96.

Kottler, J.A. (1991) **The Complete Therapist**. San Francisco: Jossey-Bass Social Behavioural Science Series.

Lang, P. (1969) The mechanics of desensitization and the laboratory study of human fear. In Franks, C. (ed.) **Behavioral Therapy: Appraisal and Status**. New York: McGraw-Hill.

Marks, I.M. (1987) **Fears, Phobias and Rituals**. Oxford: Oxford University Press.

Mathews, A.M., Gelder, M.G. and Johnston, D.W. (1981) **Agoraphobia: Nature and Treatment**. New York: Guilford Press.

Piasecki, J. and Hollan, S.D. (1987) Cognitive therapy for depression: unexplicated schemata and scripts. In Jacobson, N.S. (ed.) **Psychotherapists in Clinical Practice: Cognitive and Behavioral Perspectives**. New York: Guilford Press, pp. 121–152.

Ross, J. (1980) The use of former phobics in the treatment of phobias. **American Journal of Psychiatry** 136, 715–717.

Schaap, C., Bennun, I., Schindler, L. and Hoogduin, K. (1993) **The Therapeutic Relationship in Behavioural Psychotherapy**. Chichester: Wiley.

Shelton, J.L. and Levy, R.L. (eds) (1981) **Behavioral Assignments and Treatment Compliance: A Handbook of Clinical Strategies**. Champaign, IL: Research Press, pp. 167–186.

Simons, A., Murphy, G., Levine, J. and Wetzel, R. (1984) Sustained improvement one year after cognitive and/or pharmacotherapy for depression. Paper presented at the **Meeting of the Society for Psychotherapy Research,** June 1984, Lake Loise.

Whaley, D.L. and Malott, R.W. (1971) **Elementary Principles of Behavior.** New York: Prentice-Hall, Inc.

Further reading

General

Hawton, K., Salkovskis, P.M., Kirk, J. and Clark, D.M. (1989) **Cognitive Behaviour Therapy for Psychiatric Problems.** Oxford: Oxford University Press.

This text explores the application of cognitive behavioural approaches to a variety of psychiatric difficulties. The chapters on principles and assessment are good introductory guides.

Scott, J., Williams, J.M.G. and Beck, A.T. (1989) **Cognitive Therapy in Clinical Practice: An Illustrative Casebook.** London: Routledge.

As the title suggests the illustrative case examples are extremely useful in this text, which addresses not only psychological problems, but also contains chapters on cancer patients, drug abusers and offenders, which will be of use to a wider audience.

Dryden, W. and Rentoul, R. (1991) **Adult Clinical Problems: A Cognitive Behavioural Approach.** London: Routledge.

This text includes chapters on schizophrenia, elders, mental handicap, and anger and violence, which further widens the field where cognitive behavioural approaches can be applied.

Ethnicity

Ponterotto, J.G. and Pedersen, P.B. (1993) **Preventing Prejudice: A Guide for Counselors and Educators.** Thousand Oaks, California: Sage.

This book contains excellent chapters on identity formation and prejudice prevention, which are of great use to practitioners, and gives an insight into differences in identity formation, which can be of use in the therapeutic setting.

Smith, P.B. and Bond, M.H. (1993) **Social Psychology Across Cultures.** Hertfordshire: Harvester Wheatsheaf.

An excellent text that helps the clinician to understand similarities and differences, which are of relevance in the practice setting. Sections on self, groups, social influence and cross-cultural contact make this an eminently useful book.

Gender

Unger, R. and Crawford, M. (1992) **Women & Gender: A Feminist Psychology**. New York: McGraw-Hill.
This text helps the practitioner to get to grips with the various factors that affect women and their psychological development and resultant problems. Chapters on the various developmental stages as well as violence and disorders make it particularly relevant.

Worell, J. and Remer, P. (1992) **Feminist Perspectives in Therapy: An Empowerment Model for Women**. Chichester: Wiley.
As well as chapters on socialisation and womanhood, this text contains chapters on transforming traditional therapeutic models through the lens of feminist practice. It includes a section on cognitive behavioural theory and the particular needs of women within the therapeutic relationship.

Scher, M., Stevens, M., Good, G. and Eichenfield, G.A. (1993) **Handbook of Counselling & Psychotherapy with Men**. Thousand Oaks, California: Sage.
This excellent text addresses the socialization of men and how this can affect the therapeutic relationship. It includes chapters on the male client/male helper and the male client/female helper. Power relationships are analysed and strategies suggested for improving the therapeutic relationship.

SECTION 3

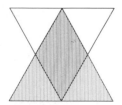

Developing Good Practice

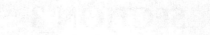

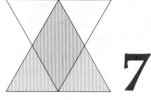 **7**

A Framework for Good Practice
Ethical Issues in Cognitive Behaviour Therapy

Althea Allison

Key issues

- The sources of moral dilemmas
- Principles, virtues and individual conscience
- Consequences, duties and responsibilities
- Relationships
- Strategies
- When things do not go as planned
- Supervision and reflection

Overview

This chapter will be concerned with the ethical and moral issues related to the practice of cognitive behaviour therapy.

The chapter is based on the premise that the value of ethical frameworks and moral codes is not founded on their ability to supply ready-made solutions to the dilemmas identified, but that guiding moral principles and virtues may help to facilitate the process of exploring 'right' decisions. It will be equally important to explore aspects surrounding the consequences of one's actions and interventions, together with the rights and duties incumbent in the professional relationship.

The individual characteristics of the professional in relation to ethical decision-making will also be addressed. Whilst many groups of professionals may use this book as a resource, special reference will be made to nurses and the particular influence of the Code of Professional Conduct of the United Kingdom Central Council for Nursing, Midwifery and Health Visiting (UKCC) (1992) on their work.

Introduction

What do you think the reply would be if each one of us was to be directly asked the question 'Do you know how to choose right actions from wrong actions?' It is highly likely that we would respond in the affirmative and may be even slightly outraged at such a question. However, that is exactly what the focus of this chapter will be: how, as professionals, do we make ethically and morally sound decisions in relation to our work with clients and, in particular, in relation to cognitive behavioural therapy?

We all make decisions about our lives, relationships and conduct for ourselves, and sometimes for those close to us. Indeed, I would guess that most of us would truly believe that we try to lead 'good' lives within our own personal sphere. Within our professional roles, however, personal yardsticks may not be sufficient, as other pressures are brought to bear on our decision making.

Professionals are faced with a large number of ethical and moral decisions in relation to client care. Such dilemmas occur on a regular basis and appear in a variety of forms. The clients may need a particular kind of help, which the professional finds personally offensive or undesirable. Professionals may be placed in a position where they may be pressured to work outside of their normal sphere of competence and responsibility. There may be conflicts of interest, employer directives or even cost implications. The list could be endless.

In responding to these dilemmas, the practitioner will draw on various resources. Broadly speaking, ethical professional behaviour will be influenced by analysis and application of moral philosophy and ethics, personal values and beliefs, the professional role occupied at the time and the professional conduct expected by society at large.

It would be easy to ignore or undervalue the ethical dilemmas involved in the delivery of cognitive behaviour therapy (CBT). After all, is it not true that all CBT interventions are aimed at improving life for the sufferer who is consulting you? How can such well-motivated intentions be ethically doubtful?

Consider for a moment the following proposition. Imagine an operating theatre, pristine and shining. There is a patient on the operating table with part of their head shaved awaiting brain surgery. The surgical team are working in unison and the surgeon raises her hand to make the first incision into the area of the brain that is responsible for personal characteristics and thinking processes. The target area has been carefully identified before the work began. When the patient on the operating table wakes up, will she still be the same person? Will the physical touching and consequent changing of the area of the patient's brain responsible for making her recognisable as the person we have come to recognise, cause changes for better or worse?

I would contend that the patient will be different because the way she thinks will be altered. The patient's individual perception and resulting behaviour will consequently be altered, and the characteristics that made them unique will now be different. They will of course be unique in a new sense. As for whether the changes will be for better or worse, then the individual assessment by the patient of the changes and the 'knock-on' effect of those changes in the patient's life will become important in the evaluation process.

So, why is this analogy with brain surgery helpful to our discussion about ethical issues in CBT? CBT is aimed at altering the thinking processes of the individual and consequently the behaviour they exhibit.

Three assumptions underlie cognitive behavioural interventions (Trower et al. 1988: 4):

1. Emotions and behaviour are determined by thinking.
2. Emotional disorders result from negative and unrealistic thinking.
3. By altering negative and unrealistic thinking, emotional disturbances can be reduced.

Although not physically touching the brain like the surgeon, CBT therapists certainly do 'touch' the brain in a metaphysical sense. This touching is directly aimed at changing the thinking processes of the person she is working with and, as a consequence, the perception of emotions and experiences will be appraised quite differently from those she has been used to doing. A success one might argue. However, the changes brought about may have consequences that are not so desirable, depending upon which player one is in the scenario.

This may not necessarily be an argument for not offering opportunities and choices for change, but it does raise questions about which choices are offered. Just as the surgeon will carefully target the area of the brain she needs to touch, then the CBT therapist will target very precisely where she will aim her interventions to bring about change. One could no doubt argue that co-operation, consent and involvement of the client in the planning are major features in the design of a CBT programme, but we will return to these arguments.

In common with other treatment modalities, CBT will sometimes be successful, sometimes not so successful and sometimes have unplanned for side-effects. Because CBT interventions have enormous potential for bringing about change it is perhaps arguably even more important that interventions are designed in an ethically sound form.

The sources of moral and ethical dilemmas in CBT

Beauchamp and Childress (1994) suggest that moral dilemmas arise when moral considerations supporting more than one course of action present themselves. The essence of the dilemma lies in the competing moral duties and obligations of the individual in relation to other persons, the community and themselves. The consequences of action or inaction may also be influential in the decision process. This may be evident where alternative treatment strategies may be viewed as equally effective but, owing to costs or contracting arrangements, decisions may need to be made with an eye to resources as the primary indicator rather than patient need.

Sometimes the laws and customs of a particular society will determine the scope of moral obligations to be assumed by individuals in that society (Gillon 1986). Although it may be fairly clear that practitioners have professional and legal obligations to others in their care, is it equally as clear that these legal and professional obligations are the same as moral obligations?

In pursuit of an answer, we may look to Seedhouse (1988), who suggests that work for health is a moral endeavour. In striving to increase the health chances of individuals in a person-centred way, then it can be seen that work for health may indeed be argued to include moral issues. An example would be respecting persons in honouring their choices to do with health or representing their health interests when unable to do so for themselves. CBT is very much person centred and is aimed at increasing the person's ability to help herself. The focus of therapy is clearly to do with increasing the mental health of individuals. As such, beliefs and ideas about what constitutes mental health need to be addressed.

As individuals, we bring our own beliefs, values and attitudes to each situation we encounter. When we meet a problem that challenges our normal way of acting, we may in the first instance look to our own personal experience and beliefs. Personal action guides may not be sufficient, however.

What place is there for differing cultural and religious beliefs within our own personal frameworks? There may or may not be a space. Will our own view of the world be influenced by gender or class? What justification is there for generalising our own view of the world to others? Perhaps more importantly, if CBT focuses on changing the frame of reference and belief system of individuals in therapy, whose frame of reference should be used?

As a member of a professional group, collective values and beliefs become influential. It may be argued that professional groups carry an added responsibility towards others by virtue of their professional role. Richman (1987) uses Barber's (1963) criteria for identifying four essential attributes of professional groups including: generalised knowledge; dedication to community interests; a code of ethics internalised by all members; and public recognition which suitably rewards their work endeavours. Richman asserts that, for professional groups, a code of ethics entails the formation of a standard of personal conduct above that of the 'rest' of society.

Professional codes of ethics include specific rules relevant to the person in the professional role. These rules specify normative standards and may apply to professionals over and above ordinary moral codes, which apply to society in general. It has been suggested that those who choose to join the nursing profession are under certain moral obligations by virtue of the profession into which they enter (Melia 1989; Chadwick and Tadd 1992).

So far, then, we can see that professionals may be faced with constraints to their practice because of influences which may be integral parts of themselves, influences which form part of the expected norms of conduct within their chosen professional group, from society as a whole and from the law.

Principles and rules

Four moral principles are frequently offered as a broad framework for aiding analysis of health care dilemmas (see Beauchamp and Childress 1994). These four principles are: respect for autonomy; beneficence; non-maleficence; and justice.

Respect for autonomy

The principle of respect for autonomy is, in essence, the requirement of one moral agent to respect the autonomy of other moral agents. It is distinguishable from autonomy, literally self-rule, which refers to the capacity to think, decide, and act freely and independently. The limitations for respecting the autonomy of a moral agent lie with the boundaries of where the autonomy of one moral agent is impinged upon by another (Gillon 1986). Often in the early stages of CBT, the therapist will lead the planning of the care programme. This can be due to the fact that the client at that time does not have a clear idea of where she most needs help or, indeed, what help she needs. Therefore, decisions made in relation to designing a care programme have implications for encroaching on the autonomy of the client, particularly where compliance is expected and where little, if any, contribution is being made by the client at that point in treatment. It underpins, therefore, the notion of informed consent to treatment and would outlaw coercion.

Non-maleficence

Non-maleficence, meaning above all do no harm, refers to the obligation to avoid bringing about harm to another. Avoiding doing harm as a prima facie duty, however, may not always be morally defensible where there is a competing opportunity to bring about good (Gillon 1986). It may be that some aspects of the behavioural part of a CBT care programme are very uncomfortable, maybe even frightening for the client. However, if a greater good can be brought about, it may be deemed acceptable to cause some suffering in the pursuit of more rewarding goals. Of course, such a decision would need thoroughly defending in terms stronger than 'Well, think how good you'll feel when you can get to the shops!' Basing decisions on the foundation that you are exercising your judgement in order to bring about a better outcome for the client may well be a paternalistic way of working and may subjugate the client's autonomy to the therapist's power.

Justice

The principle of justice is perhaps most usefully understood in relation to the allocation of resources. Rawls (1976) offers an understanding of justice as fairness. He suggests that inequality should work to the benefit of the least advantaged and that maximal individual liberty should be compatible with the same degree of liberty for everyone. Resource allocation is a common theme in the policy-making arena and has far-reaching implications for client care. An interesting example of this type of problem is illustrated by the following scenario.

A community psychiatric nurse (CPN) was requested by a local general practitioner (GP) to undertake an assessment for a young mother with two small children. On assessment she appeared to be suffering with anxiety and phobia problems. The CPN designed a plan of care based on CBT principles and returned to the GP with the assessment and the plan. The cost implications of the programme designed by the CPN were deemed by the GP to be unacceptable, given his limited resources and his need to allocate resources fairly for **all** the patients on his list. The client was offered the alternative of a prescription drug, which was said to be very effective for patients with her symptoms, and advised to join a self-help group.

These three moral principles confer an obligation on moral agents to have respect for others, not to do them any harm and to treat them fairly. Therefore, any action performed in accordance with these principles constitute acts which are in accord with ordinary moral standards.

Beneficence

The principle of beneficence requires a moral agent to promote the welfare of others but needs to be tempered by non-maleficence, where the cost may be personally too high. An obligation to act in a way that will benefit others cannot be expected if that act results in significant harm to the individual carrying out the act. Appeals to the principle of beneficence, to do good, may make a higher demand on the moral agent. For the CBT therapist, promoting the good of others may involve sharing responsibility and power in order to empower the individual.

The principle of beneficence does not require an agent to act in an heroic fashion in order to benefit others, even in an emergency situation. The ideal of beneficence, which does include an element of risk taking, may be praiseworthy but not mandatory. In addition, it may not always be clear what action is beyond a minimal requirement, yet fall short of heroism, e.g. technical competence may be an ordinary expectation of a professional, but the compassion and care that accompanies the action cannot be made mandatory. Consider the depressed person with recurring suicidal thoughts who wishes to avoid admission to hospital. This person may require an element of risk taking on the part of the therapist. The professional judgement involved in trying to design a plan of care that respects the autonomy of the individual, is skilled and caring yet, balanced against the risk of self-harm, may well call the principles of beneficence and non-maleficence into opposition.

It can be seen, then, that these four principles are both complementary and yet at the same time potentially antagonistic with each other. What they do offer the practitioner, however, is a preliminary framework or action guide from which to start analysing the ethical dilemmas with which she is faced.

Rules

Everyone is likely to be familiar with the saying, rules are made to be broken. The problem with rules is not that they are not needed at all, but that their lack of flexibility means that they cannot always be applied justly or with precision. Without some kind of rules, however, anarchy would prevail.

On a personal level, we have our own rules about how we will behave and sanctions may be applied either from within our own internal controls or by facing the consequences of our actions. On a societal level, society has rules that we are expected to observe in the interest of law and order, and democracy. Within our own groups, there will be rules, explicit and implicit that we will be expected to observe in order 'to belong'. Without some form of rules there would be very little chance of maintaining a common consensus.

Professional groups are no different. One of the ways in which we recognise a professional group is the presence of internal mechanisms for dealing with those members who break the rules. This is evident in the established professions of medicine and law, and sought after by newer professions and so-called semi-professional groups.

Several codes of ethics are available for the nursing profession. There is an international code (International Council of Nurses 1973), but there are also codes for the United States of America, Canada and the United Kingdom (Chadwick and Tadd 1992).

The UKCC Code of Professional Conduct (1992) is issued to all registered nurses, midwives and health visitors. The UKCC is the regulatory body for the nursing profession and is responsible for the maintenance of professional standards. All members of the profession are required to practice and act in accord with the standards and framework provided by the Code of Professional Conduct.

The Professional Code of Conduct (p. 2) exhorts nurses to:

> . . . act at all times in such a manner as to:
> - safeguard and promote the interests of individual patients and clients;
> - serve the interests of society;
> - justify public trust and confidence and
> - uphold and enhance the good standing and reputation of the professions.
>
> As a registered nurse, you are personally accountable [author's emphasis] for your practice. . . .

Thereafter, 16 clauses follow with clear directives related to professional behaviour and decision making for the nurse.

The Code of Professional Conduct is not an ethical code as such. However, the Code of Conduct makes appeals both explicitly and implicitly to major moral principles and professional virtues (Cain 1995). It can be shown, therefore, that there is a role for the Code of Conduct in ethical decision-making. The code has a general application, which does not remove from nurses the responsibility or capacity to make ethical decisions (Chadwick and Tadd 1992).

Whilst the UKCC Code of Professional Conduct can be used as a guide to making decisions, it does not provide clear direction with regard to making ethical decisions (Chadwick and Tadd 1992). What the UKCC Code of

Conduct is clear about is that the primacy of patient interests is the guiding force of the profession (Pyne 1988). This may be reassuring for members of the public who may be actual or potential patients, and clearly sets out a commitment to a set of ideals that are shared by the profession.

Pyne (1988) has also stated that the UKCC Code of Conduct is a weapon by which nurses can improve standards of care by exposing improper risks to patients. The code challenges nurses to make sure that patients and clients receive the standard of care they need and are entitled to. This he recognises may put nurses in conflict with those in authority.

The role of virtues

When considering the rights and wrongs of an act, or the duty or obligation attached to the act, it is easy to merely focus on the action and lose sight of the attributes of the actor.

Beauchamp and Childress (1994) argue that one or two virtuous traits do not amount to a virtuous character and identify four focal virtues including: compassion; discernment; integrity; and trustworthiness. Whilst acknowledging that these four virtues may not be the cornerstone of all professional practice, they suggest that these four virtues are useful in focusing on the character of health professionals.

However, the emphasis on particular professional virtues will alter according to the nature of the relationship between client and therapist. If the relationship between client and therapist is viewed as an equal partnership organised in contractual terms, the virtues required will have a different emphasis than if the relationship is viewed as a dependent, paternalistic partnership.

The way in which therapists view themselves and their role will also call on particular virtues to be displayed. For example, in recent years, an argument for nurses to act as an advocate for their clients has been made. This would require the nurse to strongly exhibit such virtues as courage, tenacity and fortitude. This kind of requirement may be quite daunting for the nurse fighting for resources to meet the client's needs or trying to enlist the support of family members to support client progress.

A moral virtue is a character trait that predisposes the moral agent to act in accord with moral principles, rules or ideals. Such virtues may be acquired as habits or be exhibited in a disposition to act in a way that is morally right or praiseworthy. It could be argued that virtues should take precedence over action guides in ethical decision-making. When individuals are faced with ethical dilemmas, the role of ethics is to help to identify the moral principles or rules that will inform the duties, expose the possible consequences and help to identify the desired actions in that situation. In terms of character traits, a virtuous character is internal to the person and does not rely on rules to guide right actions. Indeed, we have seen that principles require judgements to be made particularly where those principles are in competition with each other.

It is arguable whether rules and procedures always produce a better decision than the use of these virtues by an individual. The problem in this approach is that persons of good moral character sometimes fail to discern what is right action. Indeed, recognising that there is no obvious answer may be part of the moral strength of that person, consequently discussion of principles in exploring dilemmas becomes important for identifying the morally good action.

A desire to do what is right is fundamental to right action. However, if the desire is an inclination to act in a morally correct way, then it still remains important to be able to decide independently what makes a right action. A moral agent may not always perceive what ought to be done or may indeed lack the necessary virtues to carry the action through. Even where there is no lack of personal incentive and opportunity to do good, there will be occasions where people are tempted not to act in a morally good way.

Virtue and desire to do good may not be sufficient, therefore, for the moral life but they cannot be ignored as being important influencing factors in determining right action. To act in accordance with duties and obligations requires that the individual desires to do so and has a disposition to conduct herself in accordance with those duties and obligations. The consequences of action or inaction will in turn be influential in discerning right action, but will still rely on the desire and the will to act in a morally good way.

The role of conscience

A moral agent may appeal to her conscience in deciding whether or not an action is a right action. An appeal to conscience recognises the fear of loss of integrity for the individual if she is required to act or omit to act in a certain way. Generally, such a claim will be a prospective claim about how she will feel if she commits or omits a particular act, resulting in guilt and shame. As a consequence, a personal harm will be brought about. Such claims are based on the moral standard of the individual and concern a person's own acts and omissions. It is not possible logically to justify the actions of another person by a claim to one's own conscience. Therefore, to try to influence the action of another moral agent, it is necessary to invoke the principles and rules that influence an individual's conscience. An example would be a situation where an individual requires other moral agents to act or not act in a particular way, because to do otherwise would offend the conscience of that individual. This is evident where vulnerable individuals are exposed to manipulation. An appeal to stop such behaviour because it offends the conscience of an individual may suffice for them, but appeals to principles and rules such as, above all avoid doing harm to others would hold much more value in trying to alter the behaviour of others.

An appeal to conscience, of course, is maximally autonomous, but cannot stand alone in influencing standards of behaviour. A state of conscience comes about following reflective thinking on a previous experience, present circumstances and future conduct, considered in relation to the individual standards held. A moral agent may decide an action is wrong because it is prima facie wrong, e.g. not taking life, not telling the truth, not breaking promises. Where such imperatives cannot bring about a clear direction for actions or inaction, then it is the significance of the moral judgement related to supporting principles and rules that influence the conscience of the individual. Conscience can be seen then as one tier of moral justification (Beauchamp and Childress 1994).

An agent's conscience may cause difficulties in relation to the actions of others as well as themselves. This may be experienced especially where she has been delegated to perform an action or is required to refrain from an action. It may be that the agent can deal with this from an individual perspective by performing or not performing the required action, but this may not be enough if the individual believes that fundamental and universal duties are being violated.

At a team meeting, where referrals were distributed and discussed following assessment, a client who had been suffering from anxiety and drink-related problems was presented to the group. On assessment it had been discovered that the client required a fairly long-term plan, owing to the emergence of a very complicated situation. The client's assessment uncovered unresolved grieving and marital problems in addition to the primary reasons for the referral. The therapist was told that, owing to the pressure of new referrals on the waiting list, a maximum of six sessions were to be utilised for the care programme. The therapist was advised to work only on those aspects of the client's need that could be dealt with in that time scale.

The therapist complied and fulfilled the required function in as thorough a way as possible, but the therapist was still left with personal feelings of unease about the quality of the care delivered to the client and the deficits in the programme.

So far, we have considered the use of guiding rules and principles to be applied when endeavouring to bring about right action. The importance of the personal characteristics and virtues of individual moral agents in effecting right action have also been addressed. The role of conscience for the moral agent has been examined in the context of ethical decision-making.

We can now see that, in seeking right action through recourse to action guides and the inherent goodness of individuals, we may be left wanting. Consideration of the consequences of action or inaction, together with the context in which the dilemma occurs are all worthy of consideration in seeking a right decision. Increased responsibilities ascribed to individuals within a professional role will be discussed later in the chapter.

Applying an ethical framework to CBT

We have now arrived at the point where it is possible to look more closely at the practice of CBT and try to elicit where the ethical and moral considerations we have reviewed may be specifically helpful.

Managing the client–therapist relationship

CBT is negotiated and delivered through the medium of a therapeutic relationship. Therapeutic relationships are fraught with ethical dilemmas. Let us explore briefly what a therapeutic relationship is and why it is prey to ethical dilemmas.

A professional relationship is a therapeutic relationship not a social relationship. What is the difference? Within a social relationship, the needs of both parties will be met, whereas within a professional relationship, the needs of the client will always be the focus of the relationship. This automatically alters the balance in the relationship from one of equal consideration to one where the professional must always be vigilant to the needs of the client. As a result, the professional relationship is deliberate and planned whilst a social relationship will be more spontaneous. The boundaries of acceptable disclosures will also be altered within a professional relationship. Restraints which may operate in a social environment will not operate within a professional relationship. It may be that the client will be encouraged to express feelings and thoughts that are not acceptable in the social setting, and may even cause the professional some personal discomfort. Both the therapist and the client enter the relationship as strangers not friends, and it is incumbent on the therapist to maintain an appropriate focus for the relationship, separating the therapist's personal needs from those of the client.

The spontaneity and ease of the social relationship usually signifies that the people involved respect and like each other. Whilst within a professional relationship, it is unfortunately true that it is not always easy to like one's clients.

An example from practice would be working on anger management with a person who has a history of beating people up. The ability to empathise and accept the client openly and without judgement may be sorely restricted.

In order truly to respect the autonomy of the client, it is necessary to accept the person unconditionally. This means to respect the other person as an equal, without censure or judgement. Clients generally become clients because they have a need which can be met (at least theoretically!)

by the therapist. This immediately puts the client in a position of dependency. As a result, the client finds themselves with little choice but to place their trust in the professional.

Trust is a further component of the therapeutic relationship that may hold hazards for the practitioner. Willingness to enter into a trusting relationship with a professional will be influenced by how the professional's character is perceived. In order to place trust in another person, one must have confidence in them, to be secure in the knowledge that they will act in a particular way. Trust entails vulnerability and placing oneself into the hands of someone else. A person is trustworthy if they can be counted upon not to betray that trust.

We can now consider more clearly how recourse to virtues may help in analysing the ethical and moral dilemmas the therapist faces in practice.

The fiduciary relationship

Bayles (1989) emphasises a professional's special obligations to be worthy of client trust. It would be hard to disagree with this claim. Bayles argues that professional conduct can be informed by the demands of a trusting fiduciary relationship. The sense of trust referred to is not a paternalistic trust where a professional is left to make decisions for the patient without consultation. The interpretation of trust offered is a trust that fulfils the functions for which the professional has been engaged and a trust which gives the client what they want. In addition, a trustworthy person will display a character that includes several virtues. A good professional, he contends, is honest, candid, competent, diligent, loyal, fair and discrete. These characteristics are offered as virtues that a trustworthy professional possesses but it is suggested that the obligations contained in these requirements can also be viewed as norms of conduct. As such, the professional is presented with certain responsibilities and duties that must be honoured. However, even though the therapist may possess the character traits described, this does not necessarily mean that the fulfilment of the responsibilities will necessarily follow.

It is important to remember here that the therapist is also engaged in a trusting relationship with their employer and possible conflicts of loyalty may present themselves which cannot be resolved by looking to virtuous conduct alone.

It may be useful at this point to explore the impact of the implied responsibilities and duties to which Bayles (1989) refers on the practice of CBT.

Honesty

At face value, being honest implies not stealing, not lying and not cheating. By implication the professional who does not observe the obligation to avoid these behaviours is not worthy of client trust. However, it is frequently possible for the professional to find themselves in a situation where it is tempting to justify such behaviour. Take the obligation not to steal from clients. Obviously this would include things such as money and goods, but there are other less tangible things that can be stolen from clients. When deciding how much time to spend with particular clients, it is possible that the relationship the practitioner has with the client may influence how much time is allocated or not allocated as the case may be. A client whose company is enjoyable, or whose home is more clean and comfortable, may receive more than their fair allocation of time at the expense of a less attractive client. Consideration of the principle of justice would be significant in deciding how to organise time.

Failing to provide a service can also involve dishonesty. We may argue that the responsibility of the professional in CBT is to assess the needs of the client, design the plan of care and deliver the means to achieve success. Resource limitations and policy directives that are external to the therapist may affect their ability to meet needs. At what point is it the responsibility of the professional to challenge external influences on care delivery? The example of the CPN referred to earlier is significant here.

Clients can also suffer from being robbed of their respect. It is impossible always to like everyone. Sometimes clients do not make the progress we would have liked them to make and that is frustrating. Where there are difficulties experienced with clients it is tempting to 'let off steam' in a disparaging manner to other colleagues. This diminishes the client and treats them without the respect to which they are entitled. It would also constitute a breach of confidence as the client is entitled to expect that information regarding their progress or lack of progress is not discussed with other people outside of the therapeutic dimension. Exploration of feelings of frustration within clinical supervision is quite different from exasperated gossiping!

The obligation not to lie, or stated more positively, to tell the truth links with the requirement to be candid.

Candour

Whilst truthfulness involves being honest and not telling lies, candour implies volunteering information. It is possible, for example, to avoid telling a lie by not saying anything at all. If the relationship with the client is truly a partnership based on the fiduciary principle rather than a paternalistic dependent relationship, it falls to the therapist to negotiate and confer with the client on all aspects of care planning and intervention. This will entail being honest about what can and cannot be achieved, but will also require that the therapist volunteers information that may be influential in the decisions the client makes. In other words, to make a truly informed decision about treatment, the client must be in possession of sufficient information to formulate a choice. They may not always know which questions to ask and it is incumbent on the professional to anticipate and provide relevant information.

Changes that are possible with CBT may be sought after by the client but also hold wide implications for significant others in their lives. The client may not realise this at the outset of the programme. The following example illustrates this point.

A woman of 30 came to see a cognitive behaviour therapist specifically to undertake some work on assertiveness. Her agenda was that she wanted to become more assertive in order to help her cope better with workplace stresses. She was unmarried and lived with her parents in the family home. Her parents made high demands of her and expected considerable support from her. She rarely went out socially and, although she had had male friends in the past, she did not have a partner at that time. She was very committed to the programme and she became more able to be assertive at work. She also saw opportunities for change within her home life, which ended in great unhappiness for her parents, who viewed the changes in their daughter's behaviour as undesirable. The client, however, was very pleased with how she was now conducting her life and viewed the programme very positively.

Competence

Professionals are expected to be competent in the work they do. Indeed, there is an ethical responsibility to be competent to deliver the service the client is seeking. At the very least, the principle of non-maleficence, above all does no harm, should be a guide to deciding when the professional is out of their depth. There is an expectation in professional codes of practice that professionals will only undertake work in which they are competent. It is not always explicit within professional groups that updating of competence should be a continuous practice. Within the nursing profession, the commitment to competence in practice is made explicit within the Code of Professional Conduct (1992):

- Clause 3 requires nurses to maintain and improve their own professional knowledge and competence.
- Clause 4 requires nurses to acknowledge any limitations in knowledge and competence, and to decline from undertaking duties and responsibilities which they cannot fulfil with skill and safety.

What implications are there for the practitioner who is seeking to become competent in CBT? It is necessary to work with clients in order to become competent. Indeed, people using this book will be in exactly that position!

Whereas earlier in this section honesty with clients was referred to, honesty with oneself is indicated here. The desire not to lose face, not to appear unskilled and ill at ease may make it tempting to 'carry on regardless'. The qualities involved in self-awareness, in being able to recognise one's own deficits and needs, is an essential requirement of the professional in assessing her own level of competence.

However, this is not the end of the line. Once those deficits in competence have been recognised, energy needs to be spent in meeting those needs. For the cognitive behaviour therapist, clinical supervision will always be a requirement in maintaining clinical standards. For the CBT trainee, it is also the process through which the skills can be learned, modified and perfected whilst protecting the interests of the client.

Diligence

Diligence is closely associated with competence. Diligence requires the professional to deliver competent care with full commitment. For example, I have referred to time as a commodity that may cause problems of fairness for the professional. Given that lack of time appears to be a common complaint of many professionals, balancing high-quality care within the constraints of time may be problematic. If the therapist is to deliver good-quality care to each client, with enthusiasm and commitment, there are implications for the size of the caseload and the management of each client's needs.

Clients are owed a duty of care as soon as the therapist has entered into an agreement with the client. Lack of diligence may be implied where claims of negligence are made. Therapists are not infallible. Plans do not always work out as we would have wished. When things go wrong in treatment plans, one of the ingredients that may be missing is diligence on behalf of the therapist. Whilst it is tempting to lay the cause of failure at lack of commitment and insight from the client, it may on reflection be more to do with the lack of enthusiasm and support of the therapist. On a more serious level, the excuse for lack of diligence may merely disguise the lack of commitment on behalf of the therapist.

Loyalty

Loyalty implies an allegiance to the client in a therapeutic relationship. There are limits to the depth of loyalty that clients may rightly seek from professionals. The professional has a responsibility to themselves and other third-party interests to consider. Earlier in the chapter it has been suggested that demands to respect the autonomy of the individual are required to be observed only in so far as the autonomy of one person does not impinge upon the autonomy of another. If in respecting the client's autonomy the demand for loyalty to the client exacts too great a price from the professional, then the professional must decide how far to promote the well-being of the client (beneficence) and to temper any actions by minimising harm (non-maleficence).

For the nurse, this is extremely problematic as the Code of Conduct makes it very clear that the primacy of patient interests takes precedence. In our example of the client offered tablets instead of a course of CBT, it could be argued that the nurse should 'stand by' the client and not allow the client's best interest to be ignored. After all, CBT is not a palliative treatment, it offers the client a way of taking hold of her life, of bringing about changes to improve their mental health in the here and now. It also equips her with the means to maintain and improve her mental health status. A prescription may offer relief now, but it does not offer long-term gains and may even present future problems.

A further consideration of the role of loyalty for the professional relationship is in the commitment to keeping confidences. An implied contract within the therapeutic relationship would include a commitment to confidentiality for the client. The expectation that confidences will be kept may become problematic where team work is involved and where the client has made it clear that they wish personal information to be kept private. A less common but nevertheless important occasion when keeping confidences is called into question arises when third-party interests occur. For most of us, sharing information related to clients on a 'need to know basis' is a useful yardstick, together with establishing clear ground rules at the outset of therapy regarding what information can and cannot be shared. Third-party interests are addressed within the Code of Conduct (clause 10) and are, of course, dealt with in the law. We shall return to confidentiality.

Discretion

Whilst most professionals have a clear understanding of what constitutes confidential information, discretion is not so widely understood. Discretion, as Bayles (1989) points out, is a broader concept than confidentiality. Whereas confidentiality generally covers factual information gleaned from a client, discretion refers to a wider consideration of privacy.

It was not unusual for one therapist to visit a local market during Friday lunchtime to do some shopping. Neither was it unusual to meet clients who were doing the same. One Friday the therapist met a female client who was with an older woman whilst shopping at the same stall. The therapist smiled and said hello and made an innocuous comment about the weather. The client replied 'Do I know you?' and accompanied the remark with frantic non-verbal cues which the therapist took to mean she did not wish to be recognised at that moment. The therapist laughingly apologised and said she had mistaken the client for someone else. In a subsequent appointment the therapist discovered that the older woman had been the client's mother who knew nothing about her difficulties and that was how she wished it to remain.

Discretion would also include not discussing clients outside of the therapeutic domain. It may be tempting to remark on the attractiveness of a client's car or clothing, or their talents. Such disclosures may not break a confidence as such but they do intrude on the client's privacy.

Fairness

The principle of justice has been explained as fairness. The virtue of fairness therefore implies an impartiality towards clients. If discrimination is to be avoided, consideration of race, religion, ethnic origin and sex should not be influential. Less obvious traits may offer the means to discriminate, however. Unpopular clients may not receive the same consideration and commitment as those who are found to be more attractive or better company. It may be that the grounds for discrimination may not be immediately overt and may have their foundations in the therapist's personal experiences.

During a supervision session, a therapist was discussing blocks to progress with a client whose excessive drinking patterns and violent behaviour were associated with his maladaptive thinking about the causes of his behaviour. The failure of the client's business had brought about an exacerbation of the excessive drinking and consequent violent behaviour towards his partner. The man complained that the failure of his business was the fault of his partner as it was the pressure to earn more money and provide a high lifestyle which had made him take the chance of becoming self-employed and giving up a secure job. He was not willing to see other explanations for the failure of the business, such as the economic environment, market forces or even lack of business experience. Everything was the fault of his partner. He was also being non-compliant with tasks that he had been set and the therapist wanted to abandon the case.

During the session, the clinical supervisor began to pick up feelings of anger towards the client and lack of commitment to continuing the programme. After some careful and skilful probing, it transpired that the therapist could not disassociate him/herself from feelings which remained unresolved from a personal experience of dealing with problem drinking and violence.

Fairness then is particularly important for professionals who are dealing with vulnerable groups. Attention to internal barriers to fairness as well as external barriers are vital if clients are to be treated equally.

Within this section, we have pursued the norms of conduct expected of a professional within a fiduciary relationship, using Bayles' (1989) template of the professional virtues a practitioner can be expected to display.

Strategies employed in the conduct of CBT

Hawton et al. (1989) suggest that at the commencement of treatment, the assessment interview plays a significant part in the treatment plan. The main goal of the cognitive behavioural assessment is to agree a formulation of the problems and create a treatment plan in conjunction with the patient.

CBT prides itself on the use of scientific enquiry in establishing the needs of clients (gathering data) and formulating a hypothesis (naming the problem). If professionals are to exhibit true respect for persons from the outset of treatment, then consent to that treatment must be obtained.

We can define the principle of autonomy as the freedom to decide our own goals and act in accordance with those goals. We have previously acknowledged that respect for autonomy is an important moral principle. In relation to the doctrine of informed consent, the principle of autonomy is a key principle (Faulder 1985). It is therefore incumbent on the therapist to explain the philosophy underpinning that treatment and make clear what is involved in the treatment plan. Of course this entails observing the principle of veracity (being honest) with the client about the limitations as well as the possibilities of treatment.

The first strategy in CBT, therefore, is perhaps enlisting the informed consent of the client in order that the client may decline treatment if they so wish.

Once consent has been obtained and the assessment undertaken within the boundary of a therapeutic relationship, strategies for bringing about change need to be addressed.

Giving clients control over parts of their treatment and facilitating insight into the origins of their problems is empowering and mindful of the requirement to respect persons. Sometimes, however, it falls to the therapist to lead the client in a direction that may be unpleasant. Clients have frequently utilised the strategy of avoidance in coping with their symptoms. Part of a treatment regime may therefore include exposing a client to situations that are positively distressing. Does exposing the client to such unpleasant experiences constitute causing a harm? What constitutes a harm? Is causing emotional turmoil a harm? The therapist may argue that the intention is to bring about a greater good for the client and, therefore, the principle of non-maleficence is superseded by the principle of beneficence.

Homework is a key strategy in CBT. Various tasks may be set as homework depending on the client's needs. Where the client is responsible for their own monitoring and recording of information, this may be considered empowering and respectful. There are times, however, when the therapist may need to enlist the help of third parties, a spouse, for instance. Take the need to monitor handwashing behaviour. It may be that an independent player may be able to give a more accurate account of the ritual involved in the behaviour, but how far can it be justified to involve non-professionals in the care of the client? How much information is it legitimate to divulge to a third party in order to involve them sensibly in care? Is a spouse entitled to information regarding their partner's well-being? In the first instance, we would probably reply that, if the client can give informed consent to be involved in treatment, she can certainly be asked to give consent to involve others. However, a disempowered person may be further disempowered by placing them in a position of dependency and inequality.

Occasionally, the therapist must make a decision to choose a strategy that allows them to act in the patient's interest, in effect, to act in a paternalistic manner. How can such an action be squared with treating clients as equal partners in care? Sometimes the ability of the client to make autonomous choices is impaired by the emotional suffering she is experiencing and consequently her judgement may be clouded. It, therefore, falls to the therapist to use her professional judgement and act in the patient's best interest. To decide what is the patient's best interest requires that the therapist returns to independent criteria for making morally good choices on behalf of another. Recourse to principles, professional rules and a disposition to act in accordance with the guidance offered by appeal to these tools will be helpful until the client is sufficiently in control to begin to make decisions for themselves once more. This is entirely in keeping with the CBT model of the therapist having greater influence over the programme of care at the commencement of treatment, equipping the client with insight into their problems, facilitating the means to improve their situation and terminating the relationship with the client fully leading the decision-making process.

Evaluation measures are important in being able to recognise when treatment has been successful. However, even evaluation measures are not without problems. The therapist is likely to argue that they would choose independent objective measures to evaluate care. Each measure will be aiming for a particular outcome, which should have been negotiated. How can we be sure whose goals are being set? Whose measure of success will be used? Whose needs are the primary needs being met?

The following case history offers an illustration.

A couple were referred to a CBT therapist for help with sexual problems in their otherwise very happy partnership. The husband complained that his wife suffered from a lower sex drive than he did and that the problem was hers. The therapist was able to help the husband see that it certainly was a problem which he shared with his wife and that his co-operation would be very important.

It transpired that the wife had a mildly anxious disposition, a very poor self-image, was not happy with how her body looked and felt embarrassed about her shape during their physical relationship. She believed that her husband would interpret her reluctance as shyness and would find her attractive because of her shyness. His consideration for her feelings, however, meant that he stopped approaching his wife and she was confirmed in her low self-esteem, which had started to make her feel depressed. She believed she must be a bad wife because 'it was her fault'. Conversely, she also wanted to have intercourse with her husband more often but she believed that it was not acceptable to make advances to her husband, partly because of her background but also due to the false belief that her husband would not find her physically attractive unless she added some mystique to herself which she chose to do in the form of shyness and appearing demure.

Over the months, the therapist helped her focus on the maladaptive thinking about herself, the effect this had on how she presented herself and the subsequent adverse effect on her relationship with her husband. Behavioural parts of the therapy included expressing her needs more clearly and honestly with her husband regarding their physical relationship. Things progressed very well for a while. The wife became much more confident in her daily interactions and much more assertive about her needs and desires. However, the therapist received a request from the husband for an individual appointment where it was subsequently revealed that now he could not cope with his wife's sexual demands and that therapy had turned her (in his words) into a 'vamp'!

How far is it possible to evaluate the success of therapy in the scenario just described? Depending on where you stand, the assessment is likely to be quite different. As the therapist has been instrumental in bringing about these changes, is the therapist responsible for the consequences?

When things do not go as planned

In all encounters with clients, there will be occasions where the plan of treatment will not have been successful or perhaps not as successful as was originally hoped for. What ethical problems if any does this leave us with? In the first instance, if we recall the duty to act with diligence and competence in our work, it may be that we can truly say that these obligations were met and that the therapist does not carry any culpability for the lack of progress and the consequences of that result.

However, the competent practitioner will address the reasons for lack of success in a framework that encourages growth and development. Clinical supervision is, of course, the ideal place for this professional growth to occur. We can say then that, out of a less than satisfactory outcome, something good can be retrieved.

Let us consider a slightly different situation where progress does not seem to be happening. It may be that lack of progress is the result of the therapist being 'out of their depth'. Of course, this can happen to even the most experienced practitioner, but recognising the lack of expertise and seeking the appropriate guidance or further referral point would be the most ethical course of action. This may be a real challenge for the practitioner in having to admit to a lack of certain professional expertise but it would be difficult to defend any other course of action. High levels of self-awareness are demanded of the practitioner who strives to maintain high ethical standards.

For some patients, the decision to discontinue treatment may have to be considered. Occasionally this a *fait accompli*, where the client stops their involvement in therapy. On other occasions it may be the therapist who decides that the investment of time and expertise with a particular client is no longer justifiable. Here, the therapist will have recourse to the principle of justice to help to ascertain that the decision is being made fairly. Damage limitation may also be an option where there appears to be an unplanned for consequence to treatment.

Take, for example, the client who suffered with a series of phobias, which seriously curtailed her ability to conduct a normal life. As she began to gain control of her life, her partner left her. He later disclosed that he had only stayed with his partner because of her dependence on him. Now that she was able to take responsibility for herself, he no longer felt a sense of guilt for wanting to leave her and felt absolved from the obligation to 'look after her'.

Clinical supervision

More than once I have referred to the value of using clinical supervision within the practice of CBT. One value of clinical supervision is that it offers a medium to explore morally right actions and decisions as well as offering a strategy for professional growth and development in technical and educational terms.

Of course, clinical supervision is a relationship which aims to nurture growth and development in the practitioner. As such it is difficult to show where the differences with a therapeutic relationship with clients differs, if indeed it does. However, within this relationship there are rights, duties and obligations on both the supervisor and supervisee (Butterworth 1995). I would contend that the previous discussions in relation to therapeutic relationships with clients highlight the same moral concerns for consideration in the clinical supervision setting and therefore do not need reiterating here.

Clients are frequently asked to record their experiences so that the information can be used to 'move them on' in therapy. Nurses, in particular, are encouraged to keep a professional journal in order to enhance their practice. The CBT therapist should find little difficulty in using this method to enhance her own performance!

Accountability and responsibility are clear requirements for all nurses. The code of professional conduct leaves no room for doubt about the requirement of nurses to meet a particular standard in their dealings with clients. The nature and conduct of CBT encourages a mode of practice that fits firmly within these standards.

Conclusion

The first section of this chapter introduced the reader to a framework of ethical principles, rules, and virtues, which may offer a guiding influence to the CB therapist when faced with ethical decisions in practice.

The second section of the chapter looked more closely at some of the ethical issues specifically raised in the practice of CBT. This is by no means exhaustive and I am sure you will be able to identify many more. There is no finite number which can be stated in relation to ethical dilemmas. The situation changes all the time.

In so far as changing situations go, some recognition of the current changes in health care practice are implicitly alluded to.

Finally, in an attempt to bring together the entire content of this chapter, I have tried to create a visual picture, which will tie all the points together. It will help at this point to study Figure 7.1 for a few moments.

The felled tree trunk allows us to see the concentric rings which make up the sturdy tree. Each ring adds to the strength of the tree. The central ring represents us, as individuals, with our own value systems and

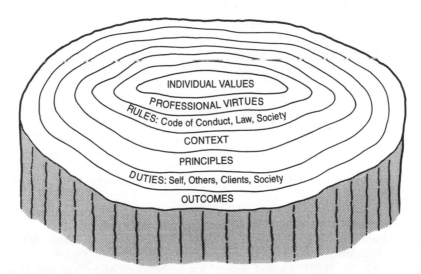

Figure 7.1 Visual representation showing the many influencing factors to be considered in making ethical decisions.

beliefs. We make up the core. The next ring represents the individual in a professional role, displaying the virtues required of the professional. The third ring represents the rules we are required to abide by, within our profession [Code of Conduct (UKCC 1992), Exercising Accountability (UKCC 1989)], within the law of the land, within society. The next ring takes account of the context in which ethical dilemmas occur and in which they must be resolved. The fifth ring offers us major moral principles to guide our analysis of the situation. The sixth ring reminds us of the duties we may be expected to honour. The final ring directs us to look towards the consequences of our actions.

The rings of the tree contribute to the strength and tenacity of the tree to withstand inclement weather and disease. When the tree is whole, it bears fruit. When the tree becomes damaged in some way, so that the rings are interfered with, the fruit of the tree is impaired.

When practitioners are able to utilise the 'strengths' found in the tree trunk (metaphorically speaking, of course), then their ethical decision-making will bear fruit too.

Discussion questions

(A) Cognitive behaviour therapy has as its focus changing the frame of reference and belief system of individuals in therapy. What are the ethical considerations that a practitioner should be aware of in enabling their clients to reframe their thoughts about the world?
(B) How may the four moral principles as described in this chapter assist the practitioner in analysing the ethical dilemmas they face during the practice of cognitive behaviour therapy?
(C) Within the context of the ethical framework presented in this chapter, how should the trainee therapist ensure that she offers her clients the duty of care they are owed?

References

Barber, B. (1987) Some problems in the sociology of professions. **Daedalus** 92, 662–673.

Bayles, M.D. (1989) **Professional Ethics**, 2nd edn. Belmont, CA: Wadsworth Publishing Co.

Beauchamp, T.L. and Childress, J.F. (1994) **Principles of Biomedical Ethics**, 4th edn. Oxford: Oxford University Press.

Butterworth, A. (1995) **Clinical Supervision in Nursing, Midwifery and Health Visiting: Development, Contracts and Monitoring.** A Second Briefing Paper, The School of Nursing Studies, The University of Manchester.

Cain, P. (1995) The ethical dimension. In Cain, P., Howkins, E. and Hyde, V. (eds) **Community Nursing – Dimensions and Dilemmas**. London: Edward Arnold.

Chadwick, R. and Tadd, W. (1992) **Ethics and Nursing Practice**. London: Macmillan.

Faulder, C. (1985) **Whose Body Is It?** London: Virago.

Gillon, R. (1986) **Philosophical Medical Ethics**. Chichester: Wiley.

Hawton, K., Salkovskis, P.M., Kirk, J. and Clark, D.M. (1989) **Cognitive Behaviour Therapy for Psychiatric Problems – A Practical Guide**. Oxford: Oxford University Press.

International Council of Nurses (1973) **Code of Nursing Ethics**. Geneva: ICN.

Melia, K. (1989) **Everyday Nursing Ethics**. Basingstoke: Macmillan.

Pyne, R. (1988) On being accountable. **Health Visitor** 61, 173–175.

Rawls, J. (1976) **A Theory of Justice**. Oxford: Oxford University Press.

Richman, J. (1987) **Medicine and Health**. London: Longman.

Seedhouse, D. (1988) **Ethics: the Heart of Health Care**. Chichester: Wiley.

Trower, P., Casey, A. and Dryden, W. (1988) **Cognitive Behavioural Counselling in Action**. London: Sage.

UKCC (1989) **Exercising Accountability – A Framework to Assist Nurses, Midwives and Health Visitors to Consider Ethical Aspects of Professional Practice**. London: United Kingdom Central Council for Nursing, Midwifery and Health Visiting, March.

UKCC (1992) **Code of Professional Conduct**, 3rd edn. London: United Kingdom Central Council for Nursing, Midwifery and Health Visiting, June.

Further reading

Downie, R.S. and Telfer, E. (1980) **Caring and Curing – A Philosophy of Medicine and Social Work**. London: Methuen.

Husted, G.L. and Husted, J.H. (1991) **Ethical Decision Making in Nursing**. St Louis: Mosby Year Book.

Mason, J.K. and McCall Smith, R.A. (1991) **Law and Medical Ethics**, 3rd edn. London: Butterworths.

Pyne, R.H. (1992) **Professional Discipline in Nursing, Midwifery and Health Visiting**, 2nd edn. Oxford: Blackwell Scientific Publications.

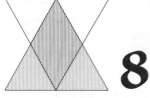 **8**

Reflecting on Your Experience and Practice
A practicum

John Turnbull and Sue Marshall

Key issues

- Improving professional practice
- Reflecting on experience
- Identifying professional strengths and needs

Introduction _____

Throughout this book we have shown how the process of cognitive behaviour therapy can bring about significant and long-lasting change in individuals, which will improve their lives. However, it should be remembered that the client is not the only person to experience change as a result of therapy. Even though we have outlined a framework of principles upon which cognitive behaviour therapy bases its approach, the uniqueness of each individual creates the need for the therapist to adapt and to learn. The motivation to rethink our practice often arises when things go wrong. This is a similar experience to that of some of our clients, who will recognise the need for change perhaps following a traumatic event or consistent disappointments. To restore our clients' confidence in themselves, we would encourage them to recognise and to learn from positive as well as negative situations. In the same way, our own personal and professional growth can only be satisfactorily achieved by a continuous reflection on all aspects of our practice and experience.

Therefore, the aim of this chapter is to explain ways in which our practice can improve through practice-based learning. A series of exercises will be presented to help you to:

- Acknowledge your current strengths and skills, and how they have been acquired.
- Recognise how current strategies you employ either aid or hinder your development.
- Devise a framework through which personal and professional growth can be encouraged.
- Recognise alternative ways of demonstrating evidence of learning.

Practice-based learning

The need for reflection can be appreciated if we examine some of the forces that are at work in the settings in which we practise. Most professionals providing health and social care today are facing increasing pressures arising from both professional and managerial influences. In reality, many of these influences will interact to generate internal and external expectations of the professional's performance.

Managerial (external) expectations

The current landscape of care is characterised by rapid changes in priorities, which frequently lead to restructuring within organisations. By simply looking back 10 years we might recognise how things have changed. There is now increased attention on health promotion, the closure of long-stay hospitals and a greater focus on primary health care. Professional attention is increasingly being drawn to clinical audit and evidence-based practice. Professionals may now be managed by people with non-clinical backgrounds as conventional career pathways have disappeared. The need to update professional knowledge and skill is now compulsory for nursing staff [United Kingdom Central Council (UKCC) for Nursing, Midwifery and Health Visiting 1992].

Professional (internal) expectations

Like the majority of care staff, professionals come to work to do a good job and expect to improve their practice with experience. Each professional would also expect his/her expertise to be more consistently applied as experience develops. This improvement will be accompanied by expectations of increased status within a service and amongst colleagues, which may be recognised financially or through increased responsibility for supervising others' practice.

Taking both sets of expectations together, we can see how there are opportunities for threats as well as challenges. Professionals will find themselves in similar situations to their clients, needing to both appraise their expectations and adjust their strategies to resolve potential conflicts. As we might well advise our clients, the key to successful coping depends on us remaining flexible.

The principal change required in our thinking is to recognise the growing importance of the workplace over theory in influencing practice development. Therefore, the professional can no longer rely on traditional courses of education as the sole means of fulfilling expectations of improvement. In fact, the focus on education rather than learning in the past has been criticised as being responsible for a separation of theory from practice.

Therefore, the practice setting must be seen as the generator rather than the receptacle of theory. Cognitive behaviour therapy has an advantage in that the components of its approach have been synthesised from the application of a range of psychological theories (see Chapter 3). This provides a useful foundation for personal and professional development, but what mechanisms exist to capitalise on this opportunity? On a personal level, what steps can you take to ensure that your own learning is maximised and that your practice can improve?

Learning now to learn

It is now recognised that prequalifying professional education cannot provide all of the experiences to develop the necessary skills and knowledge required for specialist practice. Increasing emphasis in professional prequalifying curricula is now being placed on teaching students how to learn in order that practice remains a dynamic process. A framework which is often used to encourage this to take place is the learning model first devised by David Kolb (1976) and shown in Figure 8.1. This is a relatively simple model, which encourages people to become both observers and actors within their workplace. It conceives of learning as being a cyclical process consisting of four stages, which each person must go through in order for learning to be said to have taken place. The model begins with the concrete, or 'hands-on' experience that people have and, in stage two, encourages reflection upon these experiences. Stage three occurs when people develop new hypotheses based on their observation and reflection, and stage four occurs when these ideas are tested out in practice. Once again, we should recognise that this approach is similar to

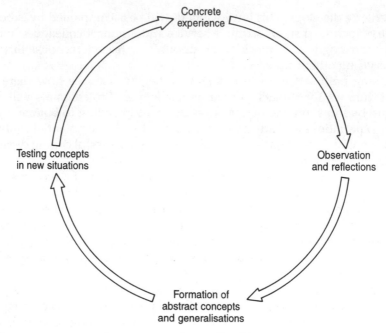

Figure 8.1   Kolb's cycle of learning.

that which we ask our clients to undergo in order to improve their own performance.

The exercises in the rest of this chapter have been designed to follow this model. As a starting point, let us look at your current job and the sorts of experiences that have brought you here.

Part one: Your experience

Activity 1

Take a piece of paper and divide it into two columns. Down the left-hand side, write down the different jobs you have had in the last 10 years. Down the right-hand side, for each job, describe the most important aspect of your development that occurred in this job and the key learning experiences that contributed to this development.

Despite the fact that we would encourage our clients to recognise their achievements, we often fail to take this good advice ourselves. We may also be guilty of seeing achievement in more conventional ways, such as examination passes or job promotion. There will be countless other examples of success, which this exercise encouraged you to recognise. Although you may have listed examples in which your development arose from educational courses you attended, we hope that your list was composed primarily of learning experiences from practice. One person completing this exercise before mentioned an example in which he had reluctantly admitted to a client that he had run out of ideas about how to take forward her care. The person was surprised at the response from the client who went on to say how 'two heads' were better than one and that they should probably sort things out between the two of them. This convinced the therapist of the need for partnership and also taught him that acknowledging what he did not know was as important as recognising the knowledge he already had. Another example came from a nurse whose work on non-verbal communication was rewarded with a comment from a patient recovering from a stroke who commented that the nurse's touch and tone of voice had been reassuring to her in the early stages of her recovery.

Comments from clients are important evidence, or testimony, to demonstrate that competence has been achieved. You might like to think of other ways in which evidence of competence could be compiled. It is often said, for example, that teaching someone else is a good way of demonstrating your own learning. This might be in the context of the supervision of others or it could take the form of a lecture or seminar led by you. If you do not get regular opportunities to carry this out, you might want to get your manager's support for doing this. With the permission of your clients, video- or audiotapes of therapy sessions can also provide evidence that learning has taken place. For some areas of competence, written evidence can be used, such as minutes of meetings or case conferences. You may have also contributed to devising policy documents, which can be used so long as you can isolate your distinctive contribution. We, therefore, need to think beyond conventional ways of compiling evidence if we are to acknowledge our own development.

We hope that these examples demonstrate the importance of the practice setting in providing evidence of learning. However, for many roles, it is equally appropriate to look beyond the job you occupy to discover how other factors in your life have contributed to your ability to fulfil your role. Skills in teamworking, problem solving, communication and negotiation skills can be enhanced by people's experience, for example, as a parent, school governor or volunteer. For anyone using therapeutic approaches, opportunities to observe other people and ourselves in a range of settings can help develop understanding and empathy.

Returning to your list, there are other factors to consider. A key point to note is whether you can detect any continuity in your development and whether you consider that your progress has been planned. We can often occupy roles without taking opportunities to discuss with our immediate managers the areas in which development needs to take place. We should not always assume that, since we have been appointed to a position, we must already be proficient in that role. It is better to look at a job as a continuum starting with being not yet competent, through competence and towards proficiency. Even then, we should look towards a new set of challenges. In this way, each individual can match his or her development needs to the demands of the role. It should also demonstrate to us that development is a continuous process and that there is no such thing as a perfect helper. Although words such as 'expert' and 'specialist' are freely used in our everyday conversations, they are misleading and potentially demotivating.

To summarise this exercise, we hope that your contribution and the text has:

- Reinforced the value of deliberate and continuous reflection on practice.
- Enabled you to recognise your achievements.
- Encouraged you to think of alternative means of compiling evidence of learning.

Your current role

Now that you have identified the achievements and areas of development that have brought you to the 'here and now', the following activity helps you to make the most of these abilities for both yourself and the clients you see.

Activity 2 (NFMED, 1992)

Now consider the role that you currently occupy in more detail. Write down your responses to the following questions:

1. In one sentence, describe the job that you do as you experience it.
2. Write down the three most important outcomes expected of you in your job.
3. List the areas over which you have control and/or influence.
4. What are the most difficult areas of your job?
5. What are the most rewarding aspects of your job?
6. How is your performance monitored?

Job descriptions are a necessary but largely unhelpful way of explaining to employees the nature of their tasks. Despite the good intentions of employers, they can limit the creativity of employees rather than encourage the type of performance that is in the interests of clients, the organisation and the individual. The activity you have just completed has given you the opportunity to construct your own role summary by looking at your job as it really is.

Being asked to summarise your role in one sentence is a challenging task. However, your answer probably included improving the lives of others, working as a team within your department and perhaps acting as a consultant on broader issues. When listing the rewarding aspects of your job, you probably thought of the benefits that you bring to your clients.

Whereas this might adequately summarise the tasks you carry out, does it really convey anything about the potential that you have to improve the lives of your clients and colleagues further? This potential may be uncovered by thinking of your role in a different way. For example, do you consider yourself a standard-setter, continually striving to improve the quality of the therapy you carry out? Could you also see yourself contributing to mechanisms by which you and your colleagues might assure minimum standards within your department? What about your role as a leader, challenging accepted views and practices, and encouraging others to think differently? Are you also an analyser or auditor, scrutinising information about your practice to create better understanding amongst others? Finally, are you exploiting your potential as a supporter of your colleagues? As we know, the nature of therapy can often make us feel isolated and the support that you expect from others is available if you can reciprocate.

If you need any further encouragement to view your role in this way, many people experience a feeling that their creativity is being stifled. This is partly because the day-to-day business of seeing clients and attending meetings allows us little time to rise above the detail of our role. However, the main barriers to innovation are the informal rules that staff create for themselves in most workplaces. A reappraisal of these expectations can lead to rapid and dramatic improvements. Continuous reflection is a means of achieving this.

Part two: Your practice

The purpose of the exercise described below is to help you to gather evidence about how you currently practise your role as a helper.

Above, in the introduction to Section 3 (p. 185) we outlined what we mean by the terms evidence and expertise. The evidence you are gathering below should relate to your current practice. In completing the first part of the exercise you should try to think about two people with whom you have recently worked. They should have similar problems or difficulties. The outcome of one should have been successful, but the other should have been less successful.

Try to choose people who you know reasonably well so that you can answer the questions in the exercise as fully as possible. When you have decided on the two people whose case histories you will use, complete the following exercise.

Activity 1

Describe in as much detail as you can the nature of the primary difficulty. That is, what was the referred problem, for example, pain management, social anxiety, reactive depression, an eating disorder? In answering this you should think about the frequency, severity, duration and nature of the problem, by asking yourself the following questions:

- How often did the problem happen?
- How long did each episode last?
- On a scale of 1–10 (with 1 being satisfactory and 10 being unbearable), how bad was the problem?
- What exactly was the problem?

Activity 2

Outline the relevant history you collected. In doing this you should focus on what you actually did, remembering that initially this exercise is about your practice prior to using this text. This activity relates to the details of the following questions:

- When did the problem begin?
- Has the problem always been as troublesome as it now is?
- Is there any family history of the problem?
- Who are the people who help the person cope with their problem?
- What efforts have been made to overcome the problem?
- Have any of these been successful?

Activity 3

What assessment tools and techniques did you use to collect your information? List the tools and techniques you used. This should include any standardised check lists, semi-structured and structured interviews with the client and any significant others, and any direct observations you make of the client.

Activity 4

What was your formulation of the problem? Remember that a formulation is a way of linking together your assessment data to help make sense of the problem of which the person is complaining. It may be that you did not complete a formulation when you worked with the people whose case histories you are using to complete this exercise. Remember the purpose of making a formulation is to help you to make sense of the person's problem and the context in which it occurs. It helps you to identify areas of work to be undertaken as therapy.

If you did not complete a formulation, then go back to Chapter 4, reread the section on formulations and try to complete one retrospectively. Below is a broad outline of what to include in your formulation. In answering the general questions below, wherever you can, think about immediate and longer-term issues.

1. Factors that are features of the environment:
   - What environment does the behaviour usually occur in?
   - Is there any kind of environment in which it does not occur?
   - Does the environment remain static during and after the behaviour has been displayed?

2. Factors that relate to the person:
   - What are significant aspects of the person's history?
   - Are there any aspects of personal style that contribute to the behaviour being displayed?
   - What social, physiological and cognitive changes occur around the behaviour being displayed?

3. Factors that relate to other people:
   - Is anyone else directly or indirectly involved in this behaviour or its consequences?
   - What is significant about this person/these people being involved?
   - Would the same thing happen if other people were involved?

4. Factors that relate to reinforcement:
   - What does the person stand to gain from engaging in this behaviour?

■ Does anyone else gain anything?
■ What features of the individual, the environment and the other people support the reinforcement value for the person?

Look back to Chapter 6 and find the case history of Jim and his wife Dorothy. Figure 8.2 shows an example of how you could represent a formulation of the assessment data. Formulations are dynamic points, which can be added to as you gather more information.

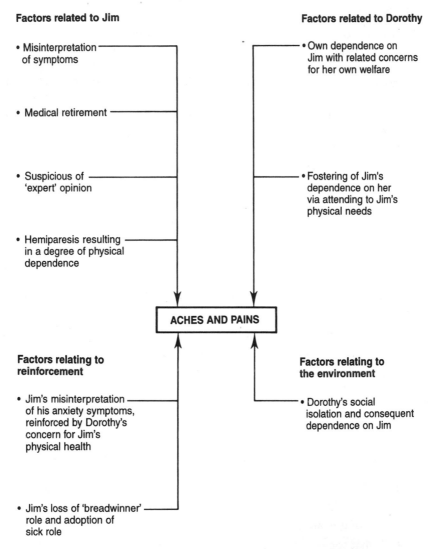

Figure 8.2   Representation of a formulation of the assessment data.

Activity 5

What were the outcomes you identified with the client? Describe the various outcomes which you and the client agreed upon. You should do this in as concrete terms as possible, identifying your criteria for success. Identify the outcomes you achieved and think about why you achieved them.

Activity 6

For those outcomes you did not achieve, list the factors that may have contributed to this:

- Factors that relate to the therapist.
- Factors that relate to the client.
- Factors that relate to other people.
- Any other factors.

Activity 7

Now go back to your description of the person's history, the assessment information and the formulation, and list any changes you would make to take account of the cognitive element of the presenting problem. In completing this you should refer back to chapters in the text that describe these aspects of cognitive behaviour therapy. You should also review your formulation with someone who has some expertise in using a cognitive behavioral approach.

Activity 8

What aspects of the unachieved outcomes could relate to cognitions of the client and cognitions of the therapist?

Activity 9

Make a careful note of what you would do differently if you were to embark upon this piece of work now. Discuss these changes with someone who is experienced in using cognitive behaviour therapy.

The exercise below is designed to take you through a short, self-directed course of cognitive therapy. To do this you need to spend some time talking to a trusted peer or supervisor about your role as a helper/therapist. The discussions should focus on the case material you have used to complete the exercise above and should allow you the opportunity to reflect on your thoughts and feelings about the work you have described above.

Activity 10

During your discussions you should note any automatic thoughts you have about being a therapist/helper. For example:

- 'I always find it hard to ask people about their relationships.'
- 'Getting the right assessment information is almost impossible during the first session – then I have nothing to use for session two.'
- 'I have never managed to work well with people who are having self-control problems.'

Activity 11

Identify one or two of these thoughts to work on, and begin by setting yourself a homework task of monitoring the frequency of this thought and the influence it has on how you feel. You should do this for a couple of weeks. In doing this you should look back at Chapters 4 and 5 for some help with constructing and keeping self-monitoring tools, e.g. diaries.

Activity 12

As you keep your diary, make a separate note of the difficulties you encounter in completing the task. This should help when you work with people who are distressed and come to you for help. Bear in mind when working with clients that their difficulties in completing the homework tasks are likely to be compounded by their presenting problem.

Activity 13

After you have completed your self-monitoring, you should begin to challenge your negative automatic thoughts by doing some reality testing, by asking yourself 'what is the evidence for this?'.

Activity 14

In addition to your reality testing you should consider what antidote thoughts you could use to challenge these negative automatic thoughts. When you do this, refer back to Chapter 5 for a full discussion of challenging negative automatic thoughts. Once again it would be helpful for your future practice to note any difficulties you experience in completing this task.

Activity 15

When you have completed this paper exercise you should try it '*in vivo*', noting the impact it has on your affect. Does it reduce your anxiety or increase your feelings of personal effectiveness? By referring to Chapter 6, you will be able to identify methods for ensuring that what you do in one setting can translate to another setting.

Part three: Your self-assessment exercise revisited

This exercise, which you may also have completed at the beginning of the book, has been prepared to give you an opportunity to reflect on your skills as a cognitive behaviour therapist. In completing the exercise, you need to be honest about your current level of competence. It is probably a good idea to discuss your response to the various questions with someone you know well and who is familiar with your clinical work.

This assessment is not a standardised tool. It is simply a guideline to help you be reflective in your practice. By completing this exercise now, you can compare it with your reflections before you read this book.

Activity 1

Think about someone you know who is an example of a competent cognitive behaviour therapist. Describe the skills and knowledge s/he has. If you cannot summarise these, then ask the person to do it with you. Try to identify which characteristics are 'skills' and which are 'knowledge'.

Activity 2

Using the list as a guide, consider which of these characteristics you currently have. On a scale of 1–10, think what you would score for each of them (1 = do not have; 10 = feel fully competent).

Activity 3

Ask a client permission to tape a session of therapy and use the tape to assess yourself on the characteristics you have identified as features of a skilled therapist. It is a good idea to use tapes as part of your supervision to help you to identify areas of strength and need in your practice.

Discussion questions

1. In what ways could an organisation be said to learn? Would you describe the service in which you work a learning organisation?
2. What are the advantages for professionals in networking? Why is networking particularly important in today's health service?
3. In what ways does clinical supervision differ from individual performance review (IPR)?

References

Kolb, D.A. (1976) Management and the learning process. **California Management Review** XVIII, Spring.

National Forum for Management Education and Development (1992) **Crediting Competence.** (Section 2.10) London: NFMED.

UKCC (1992) **Postregistration Education and Practice.** London: UKCC.

Further reading

Garratt, B. (1994) **The learning organisation** London: Harper Collins.

Palmer, A., Burns, S. and Bulman, C. (1994) **Reflective practice in nursing: the growth of the professional practitioner**. Oxford: Blackwell.

Schon, D.A. (1991) **The reflective practitioner**. 2nd edition. London: Temple Smith.

Index